Objective Tests for Nurses
Book Four

Other books in the series contain questions on anatomy and
physiology, and nursing care of medical and surgical conditions related to the
following body systems:

Book One: The structure of the body
Book Two: The skeletal-system and the muscular system
Book Three: The circulatory system and the respiratory system

Forthcoming titles
Book Five: The nervous system and the special senses
Book Six: The endocrine system and the female reproductive system

Objective Tests for Nurses
Book Four

The digestive system and the urinary system

Compiled and edited by

Janet T. E. Riddle
RGN RFN ONC RNT(Edin)
Formerly Senior Tutor, Western District College of Nursing
and Midwifery, Glasgow

With contributions from

May Lee
RGN SCM RCNT(Edin)
Clinical Nurse Teacher, Western District College of
Nursing and Midwifery, Glasgow

Christine E. Mellor
SRN RNT
Nurse Tutor, School of Nursing
Manchester Royal Infirmary

Rosa M. Sacharin
BA RSCN RGN SCM Dip N(Lond) RNT
Nurse Teacher, Western District College of Nursing
and Midwifery and Royal Hospital for Sick Children,
Yorkhill, Glasgow

Jean Till
SRN RNT
Senior Nurse Tutor, School of Nursing
Manchester Royal Infirmary

Foreword by Margaret W. Thomson
RGN RSCN RNT SCM
Chief Executive Officer to the
National Board for Nursing, Midwifery
and Health Visiting for Scotland

CHURCHILL LIVINGSTONE
EDINBURGH LONDON MELBOURNE AND NEW YORK 1982

CHURCHILL LIVINGSTONE
Medical Division of Longman Group Limited

Distributed in the United States of America by
Churchill Livingstone Inc., 19 West 44th Street, New York,
N.Y. 10036, and by associated companies,
branches and representatives throughout the world.

First published 1982

ISBN 0 443 01742 5

British Library Cataloguing in Publication Data
Riddle, Janet T. E.
    Objective tests for nurses
    Book 4: The digestive system and the urinary system
        1.   Nursing – Problems, exercises, etc.
            Title
610.73'076   RT55

Library of Congress Cataloging in Publication Data
Riddle, Janet T. E.
    Objective tests for nurses.
    Bibliography: p.
    Includes index.
    CONTENTS: — book 2. The skeletal
system and the muscular system. — — book 4.
The digestive system and the urinary system.
1. Nursing – Examinations, questions, etc.
I. Dinner, Joan, joint author. II. Title.
RT55.R52   610.73'.076   80-40910   AACRI

Printed in Singapore by
Huntsmen Offset Printing Pte Ltd.

Foreword

The process of nursing has led nurses and nurse educators to be much more aware of the need to be objective in their approach to solving problems relating to nursing care given to patients. Since the first written examination for nurses, leading to registration with the General Council for Scotland was held in 1925, the Council has endeavoured to construct a reliable means of ascertaining that candidates have reached a level of proficiency which will enable them to practise safely as Registered or Enrolled nurses.

The present system of examination consists of a written paper and a continuous assessment of proficiency in practice in the clinical areas: the former to test knowledge of facts and the understanding of the application of these facts to nursing practice, the latter to assess skills and atittudes which can more properly be assessed in a clinical setting.

The Council set up the Panel of Examiners which has given consideration to the format of the questions in the written paper and to the difficulties of their construction and marking relative to the various types.

The Council welcomed Churchill Livingstone's approach to assist in the compilation of a book which would be of interest to learners and assist them in their preparation to become Registered or Enrolled nurses. In order to encourage nurse teachers to participate in the compilation of the book, a workshop was sponsored by Churchill Livingstone under the auspices of the Department of Psychology at Moray House College of Education.

Although the General Nursing Council for Scotland has not so far included multiple choice questions in the final paper, the benefit to be gained from utilizing this book as a learning aid is to be commended. I trust that it will assist the learners to develop a questioning atittude and indeed provide some of the answers in order that they may become competent practitioners of nursing.

Margaret W. Thomson

About the series

Foreword

This series of books was devised in response to the ever-increasing demand for books which would give the nurse learner practice in answering objective tests. Each book in the series consists of questions on two body systems. Within each system the questions are split into (1) those on anatomy and physiology, and (2) those on case histories based on common disorders relating to each system.

However, the authors and publishers felt that in order to be really useful the books should be more than just a collection of questions and answers. We wanted the reader to be able to find out *why* one answer was considered right and another wrong and to understand the implications involved. For this reason the nursing care questions have been based on case histories and full explanatory answers are given in these sections.

Since we regarded the books as aids to learning and revision rather than as 'crammers' for examinations, we have not confined ourselves to the use of multiple choice questions only. Instead a variety of objective tests has been used and again it is hoped that this will make the books more interesting and useful to the reader.

The questions have been tested on different groups of nurse learners and all have been found to be appropriate. No attempt has been made to grade the questions; they have been written for the nurse learner who has completed the first eighteen months of training. All the results have been evaluated by computer and subsequently analysed and any questions of doubtful ambiguity have been omitted.

Finally we felt it to be most important that the page layout used should provide space for the reader to make individual notes against the questions. For this reason we have used a page size considerably larger than is usual in books of this type.

We would emphasize that the book should be used in conjunction with other texts. A pre-knowledge of anatomy and physiology has been assumed and for further reference the reader is referred to the books in the short bibliography all of which are published by Churchill Livingstone.

Bibliography

Bloom: *Toohey's Medicine for Nurses*
Moroney: *Surgery for Nurses*
Riddle: *Anatomy and Physiology Applied to Nursing*
Ross and Wilson: *Foundations of Anatomy and Physiology*
Chilman and Thomas: *Understanding Nursing Care*

Preface

Many nurse teachers have experimented for a number of years with different types of objective test questions. This form of examination paper is becoming more popular and there is a need to produce questions for student and pupil nurses to use for practice and revision. Most of the books of this type are geared to the needs of medical students or are American publications couched in unfamiliar terminology. This series is an attempt to produce questions for British nurses.

Although the main part of this book deals with nursing, some anatomy and physiology questions have been included. These are very basic and are aimed at testing the student's previous knowledge of the subject. The questions should be studied with a textbook on hand for reference, revision and further study.

In the nursing studies the authors have attempted to cover many aspects of nursing care and to form questions which test knowledge of facts, principles, understanding and evaluation. Each case study is followed by explanations, in some detail, of why the correct answer was selected. The student may not always agree with the answer but it should be remembered that this book is not an examination and the authors will be pleased if it stimulates further study and discussion.

As editor, I would like to take this opportunity of thanking all the contributors who are helping to complete the series. We have attempted to continue with the format as first envisaged by Miss Joan Dinner and we hope that the series will continue to reflect not only her inspiration but the tremendous amount of work she put into the first two volumes.

I would like to express my gratitude to Mrs Mary Law of Churchill Livingstone who has not only helped with the editing but has spent a great deal of time having the questions tested and evaluated. Her enthusiasm has inspired us all.

I would like to thank the nurses who took the tests, the tutors who administered them, and the members of the staff of the computer centre at Moray House College of Education who produced the results and evaluations. My thanks also go to Miss J. Ross, Dr K. Wilson, Miss A. Chilman, Miss M. Thomas, Ms N. Roper and Mr M. A. Henderson for allowing us to use some of their illustrations and to many friends who have given help and encouragement.

1982   Janet T. E. Riddle

Contents

Anatomy and physiology of the digestive and urinary systems

Multiple choice questions

The following questions (1–20) are all of the multiple choice type. Read the questions and from the possible answers select the ONE which you think is correct. You can indicate your answer by writing the appropriate letter in the right hand margin. The answers to these questions may be found on page 17.

1. The length of the alimentary canal is approximately:
   A. 5 metres
   B. 10 metres
   C. 15 metres
   D. 20 metres.

   1.

2. Which one of the following organs is *not* part of the alimentary canal?
   A. Larynx
   B. Oesophagus
   C. Pharynx
   D. Stomach.

   2.

3. Which one of the following glands secretes directly into the alimentary canal and not via a duct?
   A. Gastric
   B. Liver
   C. Pancreas
   D. Salivary.

   3.

4. Which one of the following covers the bowel?
   A. Perichondrium
   B. Perineum
   C. Periosteum
   D. Peritoneum.

   4.

5. Which one of the following regions of the abdomen does *not* contain part of the stomach?
   A. Epigastric
   B. Hypogastric
   C. Left Hypochondriac
   D. Umbilical.

   5.

6. The pancreas:
    A. contains the islets of Langerhans
    B. has a duct which carries a secretion into the stomach
    C. lies in front of the stomach
    D. secretes a digestive juice which contains insulin.

    6.

7. The lacteals:
    A. absorb vitamin A
    B. are part of the large intestine
    C. form a protective covering for the small intestine
    D. secrete enzymes.

    7.

8. The large intestine or colon:
    A. has a transverse part which lies immediately under the diaphragm
    B. has a puckered appearance
    C. is joined to the small intestine in the left iliac region of the abdomen
    D. is longer than the small intestine.

    8.

9. The colon:
    A. absorbs bile pigments
    B. absorbs fat
    C. contains nonpathogenic bacteria
    D. secretes digestive juices.

    9.

10. Which one of the following glands has a digestive function?
    A. Adrenal
    B. Pancreas
    C. Spleen
    D. Thyroid.

    10.

11. Which one of the following organs does *not* return blood to the liver via the portal vein?
    A. Kidney
    B. Rectum
    C. Stomach
    D. Spleen.

    11.

12. The liver:
    A. manufactures vitamin C
    B. stores bile
    C. stores insulin
    D. stores iron.

    12.

13. Which one of the following foods is a source of carbohydrate in the diet? 13.
    A. Cake
    B. Chicken
    C. Egg
    D. Herring.

14. Which one of the following foods is a source of protein in the diet? 14.
    A. Beans
    B. Cabbage
    C. Lettuce
    D. Turnip.

15. Which one of the following is a good source of fat? 15.
    A. Cane sugar
    B. Lean meat
    C. Walnuts
    D. White bread.

The urinary system

16. The number of nephrons present in each kidney is approximately: 16.
    A. one hundred
    B. one thousand
    C. one million
    D. one billion.

17. Which one of the following is filtered from the blood into the capsule of the 17.
    nephron?
    A. Erythrocytes
    B. Glucose
    C. Lymphocytes
    D. Protein.

18. The bladder: 18.
    A. concentrates urine
    B. manufactures urine
    C. secretes urine
    D. stores urine.

19. Normal urine: 19.
    A. contains uric acid
    B. has a specific gravity of 1050
    C. is alkaline in reaction
    D. is 70% water.

20. Which one of the following is *not* present in normal urine?
    A. Chlorides
    B. Ketones
    C. Oxylates
    D. Potassium.

20.

True false questions

The following questions (21–128) consist of a number of statements some of which are true and some of which are false. Consider each statement and decide whether you think it is true or false. You can indicate your answer by writing T for true or F for false in the right hand margin beside each statement.

21–24   The alimentary canal:
    21. is approximately 18 feet long   21.
    22. is covered with fibrous tissue   22.
    23. is made of voluntary muscle tissue   23.
    24. is lined with mucous membrane.   24.

25–28   In the development of the human mouth there are:
    25. 4 permanent canines   25.
    26. 8 permanent incisors   26.
    27. 12 temporary molars   27.
    28. 20 temporary teeth.   28.

29–32   In the mouth:
    29. carbohydrates are completely digested   29.
    30. chewing forms a bolus   30.
    31. mucus is secreted   31.
    32. peristalsis is commenced.   32.

33–36   The tongue:
    33. contains the endings of the nerve of taste   33.
    34. is attached to the hyoid bone   34.
    35. is made of involuntary muscle tissue   35.
    36. is not involved in the act of swallowing.   36.

37–40   In the act of swallowing:
    37. the soft palate rises   37.
    38. the epiglottis closes the nasopharynx   38.
    39. the larynx remains open   39.
    40. the food is propelled downwards by muscular action.   40.

41–44   The oesophagus:
    41. is a muscular tube   41.
    42. is approximately 25 cm long   42.
    43. lies behind the aorta   43.
    44. lies in front of the trachea.   44.

45–48   The stomach:
        45. is a reservoir for food   45.
        46. is joined to the duodenum at the pylorus   46.
        47. is supplied by the hepatic artery   47.
        48. secretes enzymes.   48.

49–52   The small intestine:
        49. commences where the duodenum joins the stomach   49.
        50. ends with the appendix   50.
        51. has a mucous lining covered with villi   51.
        52. is made of involuntary muscle tissue.   52.

53–56   The mesentery is a fan shaped structure attached to the posterior
        abdominal wall. It:
        53. contains lymph nodes   53.
        54. contains veins which join the inferior vena cava   54.
        55. covers the small intestine   55.
        56. is part of the peritoneum.   56.

57–60   The large intestine:
        57. is approximately five feet long   57.
        58. is composed of involuntary muscle tissue   58.
        59. has a greater circumference than the small intestine   59.
        60. has a lining of ciliated epithelium.   60.

61–64   Defaecation:
        61. is accompanied by peristaltic contractions of the pelvic colon   61.
        62. is assisted by the anterior abdominal wall   62.
        63. is initiated by distension of the wall of the rectum   63.
        64. follows contraction of the anal sphincter.   64.

65–68   The liver:
        65. contains bile ducts   65.
        66. has three lobes   66.
        67. is suspended from the diaphragm   67.
        68. receives fat from the small intestine by the portal vein.   68.

69–72   The portal circulation carries:
        69. amino acids to the general circulation   69.
        70. bile to the liver   70.
        71. glucose to the liver   71.
        72. iron to the liver.   72.

73–76   In the process of the digestion of food:
    73. carbohydrates are converted into glucose by insulin   73.
    74. glycerol is one of the end products of fat digestion   74.
    75. proteins are converted into amino acids in the small intestine   75.
    76. the end products are all absorbed in the large intestine.   76.

77–80   Fatty acids and glycerol:
    77. are absorbed through the walls of the villi into the lacteals   77.
    78. pass into the general circulation by the lymphatic system   78.
    79. provide less heat than carbohydrates   79.
    80. when normally metabolised produce acetone as a waste product.   80.

81–84   Glucose:
    81. can be stored in the muscles   81.
    82. if taken in excess is stored as fat   82.
    83. is the end product of the metabolism of carbohydrate   83.
    84. produces some of the water content of the body.   84.

85–88   Protein:
    85. can be changed into urea in the liver   85.
    86. can be used for heat and energy   86.
    87. if taken in excess cannot be used by the body   87.
    88. is necessary for the growth of tissue.   88.

89–92   Of the essential food substances:
    89. carbohydrate provides heat and energy   89.
    90. fats transport vitamin C and B   90.
    91. minerals are necessary for all body functions   91.
    92. protein is necessary for the formation of blood.   92.

93–96   Vitamins are either water or fat soluble.
    93. Vitamin A is fat soluble   93.
    94. Vitamin B is water soluble   94.
    95. Vitamin C is fat soluble   95.
    96. Vitamin K is water soluble.   96.

The urinary system

97–100   The kidneys:
    97. are approximately 6 cm long   97.
    98. are covered on all sides by peritoneum   98.
    99. are protected posteriorly by the lower six pairs of ribs   99.
    100. are enclosed in a capsule of fibrous tissue.   100.

101–104 The kidneys:

101. are made of involuntary muscle tissue	101.
102. are supplied by the renal artery	102.
103. contain lymph nodes	103.
104. have a cortex and medulla.	104.

105–108 The nephrons:

105. are microscopic structures	105.
106. are tubes closed at both ends	106.
107. consist of convoluted and straight tubules	107.
108. make up the solid part of the kidney.	108.

109–112 The function of the nephrons is to:

109. filter albumen from the blood	109.
110. filter nitrogenous waste from the blood	110.
111. reabsorb glucose and water	111.
112. excrete drugs and toxins.	112.

113–116 The ureters:

113. are continuations of the nephrons	113.
114. are muscular tubes	114.
115. commence with a funnel shaped pelvis	115.
116. propel the urine downwards by peristalsis.	116.

117–120 The urinary bladder:

117. helps to control fluid balance	117.
118. helps to support the uterus	118.
119. is completely covered by the peritoneum	119.
120. secretes urine.	120.

121–124 The adrenal glands:

121. are part of the substance of the kidneys	121.
122. have a secretion which goes into the kidneys	122.
123. help to control electrolyte balance	123.
124. have a cortex and a medulla.	124.

125–128 Micturition:

125. is the act of secreting urine	125.
126. is accompanied by contraction of the diaphragm	126.
127. is accompanied by relaxation of the bladder wall	127.
128. is a reflex action voluntarily controlled.	128.

Matching item questions

The following questions (129–170) are all of the matching item type. They consist of two lists. On the left is a list of lettered items (A, B, C etc). On the right is a list of numbered items (the questions). Study the two lists and for each numbered question select the appropriate item from the lettered list. You can indicate your answer by writing the appropriate letter in the right hand margin.

129–131 From the list on the left select the organ associated with each function on the right.

A. Mouth	129. Absorption	129.
B. Large intestine		
C. Small intestine	130. Elimination	130.
D. Stomach		
E. Oesophagus.	131. Ingestion.	131.

132–134 From the list on the left select the secretion of each organ listed on the right.

A. Bile	132. Liver	132.
B. Gastric juice		
C. Intestinal juice	133. Parotid gland	133.
D. Pancreatic juice		
E. Saliva	134. Stomach.	134.

135–137 From the list on the left select a function of each organ listed on the right.

A. Absorbs fat	135. Oesophagus	135.
B. Absorbs water and salts		
C. Has a secretion which destorys micro-organisms	136. Pancreas	136.
D. Has two distinct secretions	137. Stomach.	137.
E. Moves the food onwards by peristalsis.		

138–140 From the list on the left select a function for each part of the alimentary canal listed on the right.

A. Absorbs amino acids	138. Colon	138.
B. Absorbs water		
C. Receives pancreatic juice	139. Duodenum	139.
D. Secretes the intrinsic factor		
E. Secretes bile.	140. Small intestine.	140.

141–143 From the list on the left select a function for each organ on the right.

A. Concentrates bile

141. Gall bladder   141.

B. Removes bile pigments from red blood corpuscles

C. Secretes adrenaline

142. Liver   142.

D. Secretes an enzyme which acts on fat

E. Stores glucose as glycogen.

143. Pancreas.   143.

144–146 From the list on the left select a function for each of the substances listed on the right.

A. Assists in the production of antibodies

144. Iron   144.

B. Hardens teeth

C. Is essential for the formation of erythrocytes

145. Roughage   145.

D. Provides a moist environment for living cells

E. Stimulates peristalsis.

146. Water.   146.

147–149 From the list on the left select a food which supplies a good source of the mineral on the right.

A. Cheddar cheese

147. Calcium   147.

B. Liver

C. Haddock

148. Iodine   148.

D. Lean meat

E. Marmite.

149. Iron.   149.

150–152 From the list on the left select the deficiency disease associated with each vitamin on the right.

A. Goitre

150. Vitamin B_{12} 150.

B. Night blindness

C. Pernicious anaemia

151. Vitamin C   151.

D. Rickets

E. Scurvy.

152. Vitamin D.   152.

153–155 From the lists on the left select the statement which can be applied to each vitamin on the right.

A. Can be formed in the body from carotene

153. Vitamin A   153.

B. Can be made in the skin in bright sunlight

154. Vitamin B   154.

C. Is present in liver

D. Is very easily destroyed by cooking

155. Vitamin C.   155.

156–158 A. Helps in the clotting of blood   156. Vitamin B   156.
       B. Helps to regulate the functions of
           the nervous system   157. Vitamin D   157.
       C. Helps in the healing of wounds   158. Vitamin K.   158.
       D. Is necessary for healthy bone
           formation.

The urinary system

159–161 From the list on the left select the structures which lie in association with
       each organ on the right.
       A. Duodenum   159. Bladder   159.
       B. Fourth lumbar vertebra
       C. Sacrum   160. Left kidney   160.
       D. Stomach
       E. Symphysis pubis.   161. Right kidney.   161.

162–164 From the list on the left select the structure which is part of each organ
       on the right.
       A. External sphincter   162. Bladder   162.
       B. Medulla
       C. Neck   163. Kidney   163.
       D. Pelvis
       E. Seminal vesicles.   164. Ureter.   164.

165–167 From the list on the left select the description which applies to the
       structures listed on the right.
       A. Can contract voluntarily   165. External sphincter   165.
       B. Has a peristaltic movement
       C. Leaves the bladder at the base   166. Urethra   166.
       D. Lies between the vagina and the
           rectum
       E. Leaves the bladder at the neck.   167. Ureter.   167.

168–170 From the list on the left select the statement applicable to each structure
       on the right.
       A. Acts as a filter   168. Loop of Henle   168.
       B. Carries blood to the nephron
       C. Conveys urine to the bladder   169. Glomerular capsule   169.
       D. Lies in the medulla
       E. Secretes adrenaline.   170. Renal artery.   170.

Matching item questions using a diagram
The following questions (171–206) all consist of a diagram with parts numbered 1, 2, 3, etc. This is followed by a list of parts labelled A, B, C, etc. Look at the diagram and for each numbered structure select a name from the list of parts. You can indicate your answer by writing the appropriate letter in the right hand margin.

171–173 The organs of the digestive system
    A. Appendix
    B. Caecum
    C. Rectum
    D. Liver
    E. Small intestine.

171.

172.

173.

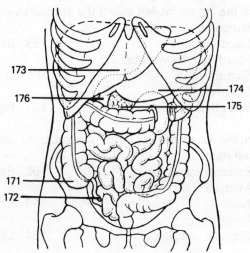

174–176 The organs of the digestive system (see diagram above)
    A. Duodenum
    B. Pancreas
    C. Pharynx
    D. Spleen
    E. Stomach.

174.

175.

176.

177–179 The mouth
    A. Fauces
    B. Hard palate
    C. Oral pharynx
    D. Tonsil
    E. Uvula

177.

178.

179.

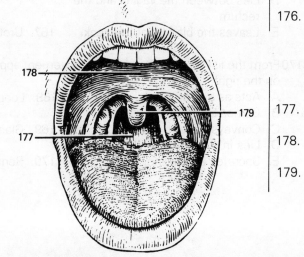

180–182 The teeth
  A. Canine
  B. Incisor
  C. Molar
  D. Premolar

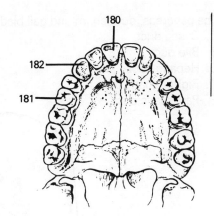

180.

181.

182.

183–185 A tooth
  A. Cement
  B. Dentine
  C. Enamel
  D. Neck
  E. Pulp

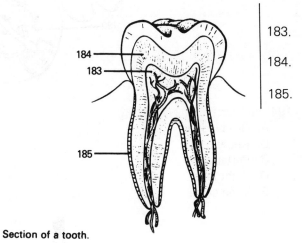

183.

184.

185.

Section of a tooth.

186–188 The stomach:
  A. Cardiac orifice
  B. Duodenum
  C. Lesser curvature
  D. Oesophagus
  E. Pylorus.

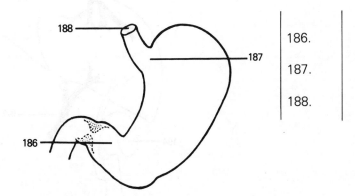

186.

187.

188.

189–191 The pancreas, duodenum and gall bladder:
  A. Cystic duct
  B. Bile duct
  C. Hepatic duct
  D. Right hepatic duct
  E. Pancreatic duct.

189.

190.

191.

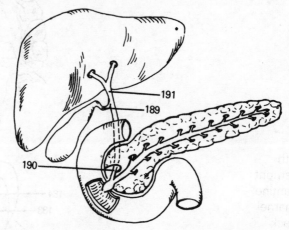

192–194 The liver:
  A. Gall bladder
  B. Hepatic vein
  C. Portal vein
  D. Right lobe
  E. Vena cava.

192.

193.

194.

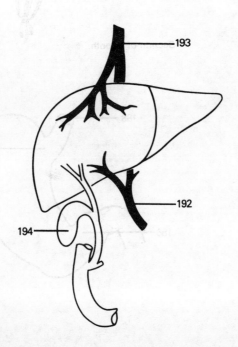

195–197 The urinary system:
  A. Aorta
  B. Renal artery
  C. Renal vein
  D. Vena cava.

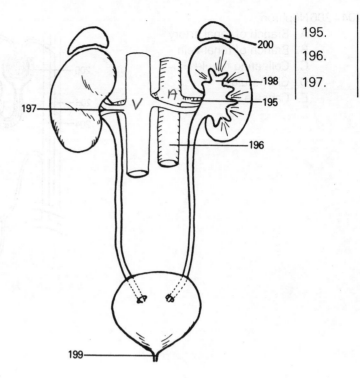

195.
196.
197.

198–200 The urinary system (see diagram above)
  A. Adrenal gland
  B. Pelvis
  C. Ureter
  D. Urethra.

198.
199.
200.

201–203 Kidney:
  A. Capsule
  B. Cortex
  C. Medulla
  D. Renal artery
  E. Ureter.

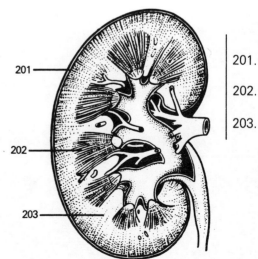

201.
202.
203.

A kidney.

204–206 Nephron:
    A. Branch of renal artery
    B. Branch of renal vein
    C. Collecting tubule
    D. Glomerulus
    E. Capsule

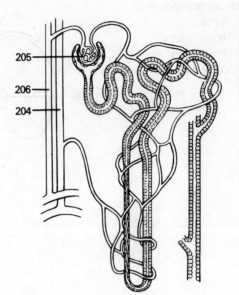

204.

205.

206.

Answers (Questions 1–206)

Multiple choice (*Page 1*)

1. B	6. A	11. A	16. C
2. A	7. A	12. D	17. B
3. A	8. B	13. A	18. D
4. D	9. C	14. A	19. A
5. B	10. B	15. C	20. B

True false (*Page 5*)

21. False	48. True	75. True	102. True
22. True	49. True	76. False	103. False
23. False	50. False	77. True	104. True
24. True	51. True	78. True	105. True
25. True	52. True	79. False	106. False
26. True	53. True	80. False	107. True
27. False	54. False	81. False	108. True
28. True	55. True	82. True	109. False
29. False	56. True	83. False	110. True
30. True	57. True	84. True	111. True
31. True	58. True	85. True	112. True
32. False	59. True	86. True	113. False
33. True	60. False	87. False	114. True
34. True	61. True	88. True	115. True
35. False	62. True	89. True	116. True
36. False	63. True	90. False	117. False
37. True	64. False	91. True	118. True
38. False	65. True	92. True	119. False
39. False	66. False	93. True	120. False
40. True	67. True	94. True	121. False
41. True	68. False	95. False	122. False
42. True	69. False	96. False	123. True
43. False	70. False	97. False	124. True
44. False	71. True	98. False	125. False
45. True	72. True	99. False	126. True
46. True	73. False	100. True	127. False
47. False	74. True	101. False	128. True

Matching items (*Page 9*)

129. C	143. D	157. D
130. B	144. C	158. A
131. A	145. E	159. E
132. A	146. D	160. D
133. E	147. A	161. A
134. B	148. C	162. C
135. E	149. B	163. B
136. D	150. C	164. D
137. C	151. E	165. A
138. B	152. D	166. E
139. C	153. A	167. B
140. A	154. C	168. D
141. A	155. D	169. A
142. E	156. B	170. B

Matching items using a diagram (*Page 12*)

171. B	183. E	195. B
172. A	184. B	196. A
173. D	185. A	197. C
174. E	186. E	198. B
175. B	187. A	199. D
176. A	188. D	200. A
177. C	189. A	201. A
178. B	190. B	202. C
179. E	191. C	203. B
180. B	192. C	204. B
181. D	193. E	205. D
182. A	194. A	206. A

Tonsillectomy

The following questions (207–248) are based on the case history given below.

Christine Foster is a 5-year-old child who lives with her parents in a modern semi-detached house on a new housing estate. Christine had been attending primary school for about 2 months when she woke up one morning and said that she did not want to go to school because her throat hurt. She looked flushed and she was reluctant to get out of bed. Her mother tried to encourage her to eat a little breakfast but to no avail. However she did drink a little warm blackcurrant cordial. She obviously had some difficulty in swallowing and vomited shortly afterwards. Mrs Foster telephoned the doctor's surgery to ask him to call and see her daughter.

When the doctor visited later that morning he found that Christine's temperature was raised and her tonsils were swollen and inflamed. He diagnosed acute tonsillitis.

Multiple choice questions

The following questions (207–220) are all of the multiple choice type. Read the questions and from the possible answers select the ONE which you think is correct. You may indicate your answer by writing the appropriate letter in the right hand margin. The answers to these questions may be found on pages 28–31.

207. The organism which most commonly causes tonsillitis in children of school age is:
    A. haemolytic streptococcus
    B. adenovirus
    C. Staphylococcus aureus
    D. Candida albicans.

207.

208. The term used to describe difficulty in swallowing is:
    A. dyschezia
    B. dyscrasia
    C. dysphagia
    D. dysphasia.

208.

209. Which of the following signs may also be present in acute tonsillitis:
    A. glossitis
    B. cervical adenitis
    C. ulcerated mucosa
    D. Koplik's spots.

209.

210. The doctor prescribed an antibiotic for Christine. The most suitable is:
    A. cloxacillin
    B. tetracycline
    C. erythromycin
    D. penicillin V.

210.

211. A suitable dosage for a 5-year-old child would be:
    A. 75 mg 6-hourly
    B. 125 mg 6-hourly
    C. 250 mg 6-hourly
    D. 50 mg 6-hourly.

211.

212. It is most important that a full course of antibiotics is given to avoid a relapse of the condition. The shortest period of treatment is:
    A. 1–3 days
    B. 3–5 days
    C. 5–10 days
    D. 10–15 days.

212.

213. In tonsillitis it is important to:
    A. encourage a good fluid intake
    B. maintain a normal diet
    C. give the child a laxative to ensure excretion of toxins
    D. give the child salt and water gargles.

213.

After two days Christine was feeling better and was able to stay downstairs on the settee for most of the day. She began to eat a little and after a week her condition was much improved. Unfortunately in the course of the next 2 years she suffered several more episodes of acute tonsillitis. During this period she often had a poor appetite and an offensive breath. On one occasion her mother had to call the doctor because Christine was complaining of abdominal pains.

---

214. In view of the medical history the most likely cause of abdominal pain was:
    A. gastro-enteritis
    B. colitis
    C. regional ileitis
    D. mesenteric adenitis.

214.

215. A loss of appetite is called:
    A. aphagia
    B. anosmia
    C. anorexia
    D. anabolism.

215.

216. The term used to describe offensive breath is:
    A. gingivitis
    B. halitosis
    C. hidrosis
    D. stomatitis.

216.

Christine's general practitioner thought it was now advisable to refer her to hospital with a view to possible tonsillectomy. An appointment was made with a consultant ear, nose and throat surgeon and Mrs Foster took Christine to his out-patient clinic. The surgeon examined her and took a detailed history. This was essential in order to assess whether tonsillectomy was in fact necessary.

---

217. Which of the following is the *least* likely to influence the surgeon in his decision to operate:
    A. frequent attacks of tonsillitis
    B. size of the tonsils
    C. loss of time off school
    D. failure to gain weight.

217.

218. In Out-Patients the sister asked Mrs Foster to assist in positioning Christine for the clinical examination. She explained that it was best to seat her facing the surgeon on:
    A. a chair with her mother standing beside her
    B. her mother's knee, while the sister restrained her hands
    C. the sister's knee, while her mother restrained her hands
    D. a chair while her mother held her head.

218.

In view of Christine's history and the clinical findings, the surgeon decided that tonsillectomy was advisable. He explained to Mrs Foster that if Christine continued to have repeated attacks of acute tonsillitis it was possible that complications such as peritonsillar abscess might arise.

---

219. Which *one* of the following is an alternative name for peritonsillar abscess:
    A. follicular tonsillitis
    B. infectious mononucleosis
    C. quinsy
    D. coryza.

219.

220. In acute peritonsillar abscess in addition to the classical presentation of acute | 220.
tonsillitis the characteristic symptom of trismus may be present. This refers
to:
   A. earache due to referred pain
   B. oedema of the uvula
   C. dribbling of saliva
   D. difficulty in opening the mouth.

At last the letter arrived indicating the date and time when Christine should report to the hospital. Her parents began to prepare her for admission.

True false questions

The following questions (221–233) consist of a number of statements, some of which are true and some of which are false. Consider each statement and decide whether you think it is true or false. You can indicate your answer by writing T for true or F for false in the right hand margin beside each statement.

221. A booklet issued by the hospital will help Mrs Foster to prepare Christine for admission.

221.

222. Children should always be told the truth about the reason for admission to hospital.

222.

223. Christine should be told that she will not be able to take her favourite teddy to hospital as there is a risk of passing on germs to other children.

223.

224. Mr and Mrs Foster should encourage Christine to talk about her admission and to ask questions about it.

224.

225. On admission a nurse should take Christine to the bathroom, wash her and put on her nightclothes.

225.

226. On admission it is most important to record Christine's temperature.

226.

227. There is a grave risk of post-operative haemorrhage following tonsillectomy if it is performed within 2 weeks of an acute inflammatory illness.

227.

228. There is less risk of bulbar poliomyelitis occurring if tonsillectomy is performed during a poliomyelitis epidemic.

228.

229. If a child of negro race is to have a tonsillectomy it is advisable to perform a sickle cell preparation test on the blood.

229.

230. If all is well, Christine's parents should be asked to leave as soon as they have signed the consent form and have answered any questions which the nursing or medical staff wish to ask.

230.

231. On the evening prior to surgery Christine should be given fluids only before settling down for the night.

231.

232. A suitable drug to use as premedication for Christine would be trimeprazine tartrate (Vallergan).

232.

Christine was prepared for surgery and was quite sleepy when the nurse and the porter took her to theatre. A tonsillectomy was successfully performed.

---

233. The best surgical method of removing tonsils is by use of a guillotine.

233.

Following the operation Christine was returned to the ward. The nurses were told that it was important to ensure that she was nursed in the correct position and that they should watch for signs of reactionary haemorrhage.

Multiple choice questions
The following questions (234–242) are again of the multiple choice type. Read the questions and from the possible answers select the ONE which you think is correct.

234. In which *one* of the following positions should Christine be nursed in the immediate post-operative period:
   A. left lateral
   B. left lateral with a soft pillow under her chest
   C. dorsal
   D. dorsal with a soft pillow under her chest.

234.

235. The *most* important observation to make immediately on return to the ward is of:
   A. temperature
   B. pulse rate
   C. vomitus
   D. restlessness.

235.

236. Which *one* of the following signs is *not* indicative of reactionary haemorrhage:
   A. increasing pallor
   B. excessive swallowing
   C. low grade pyrexia
   D. increasing tachycardia.

236.

Christine recovered consciousness soon after her return to the ward. Although she cried a little she was soon placated by the nurse who had remained with her. She settled to sleep for about an hour. Once she was fully awake the nurse gently washed her face.

237. The most appropriate care to give at this time is to:
   A. encourage the child to drink
   B. discourage the child from drinking
   C. offer ice cubes to suck
   D. offer a mouthwash.

237.

238. Observations of pulse rate should be continued:
   A. only if there is evidence of tachycardia
   B. 4-hourly for 24 hours
   C. at least hourly for the day of operation
   D. only if the child has shown signs of restlessness.

238.

239. Analgesia is not always required by children following tonsillectomy. Should it be necessary the best drug to use is:
   A. morphine
   B. chloral hydrate
   C. pethidine
   D. paracetamol elixir.

239.

Christine passed a relatively quiet night with no complications. At 6.00 am the following morning her temperature was slightly elevated. When Mrs Foster arrived the nurse reassured her regarding her daughter's condition and encouraged her to take Christine to the bathroom and then to the dayroom where she could play quietly. On return from the bathroom Mrs Foster sought out the sister and expressed concern because Christine was complaining of earache.

240. Slight elevation of temperature is:
   A. a common reaction to surgical trauma
   B. inevitable in children, due to restlessness following surgery
   C. due to mild infection which usually occurs
   D. due to release of toxins from the diseased tonsils during their removal.

240.

241. On the first post-operative day the nurses must encourage Christine to take:
   A. clear fluids only
   B. nourishing fluids
   C. a soft diet
   D. normal food.

241.

242. The most likely cause of Christine's earache was:
   A. a mild infection which often occurs following tonsillectomy
   B. fluids trickling into the pharyngo-tympanic tube
   C. small blood clots blocking the entrance to the pharyngo-tympanic tube
   D. referred pain along the nerve which serves the area from which the tonsil was dissected.

242.

Mrs Foster was encouraged to stay and participate in her daughter's care. Christine was a little miserable at times but she was obviously pleased to see her father when he arrived in the early afternoon. After his visit she settled for a short sleep, following which she seemed more cheerful. Mrs Foster encouraged Christine to eat and drink plenty of fluids which she tolerated well. An uneventful night followed and the next day the doctor said that Christine could go home. Arrangements were made and Mrs Foster was given advice about caring for Christine until she was seen again by the doctor.

True false questions

The following true/false items (243–248) refer to the advice given. Consider each statement and decide whether you think it is true or false.

243. Christine should stay indoors for 3–4 days unless it is very warm and sunny. | 243.

244. She may play with other children provided they do not have any infection. | 244.

245. If a white slough is seen over the tonsil area Mrs Foster should call the doctor. | 245.

246. Earache is always a sign of infection and must be reported immediately. | 246.

247. During the first few days it is advisable for Christine to wear a woollen hat when she goes out to play. | 247.

248. Christine should not return to school for at least 4 weeks. | 248.

Progress was maintained and Christine returned to school. During the next year her parents noticed a great improvement in both their daughter's general health and her progress at school.

Tonsillectomy answers and explanations (Questions 207–248)

207. **A** The haemolytic streptococcus is the commonest cause of tonsillitis in children of school age and in adults. In pre-school age children the causal organism is more commonly a virus (B). Staphylococcus aureus (C) causes pyogenic infection particularly of the skin. Thrush is an infection caused by Candida albicans (D) in which white spots appear on the mucosa of the mouth and pharynx but there is little inflammation.

208. **C** Dyschezia (A) means difficulty in defaecation. Dyscrasia (B) means disorder of development and is often applied to disorders of the blood cells. Dysphasia (D) means difficulty in speaking.

209. **B** Cervical adenitis means enlargement of the lymphatic glands in the neck and is usually present in tonsillitis. Glossitis (A) refers to inflammation of the tongue. In tonsillitis the tongue is furred. An ulcerated mucosa (C), which may include the tonsils, occurs in other disorders such as Vincent's angina. Koplik's spots (D) are small white spots which appear inside the cheek in the early stages of measles.

210. **D** Penicillin is the most effective antibiotic when the infecting organism is the haemolytic streptococcus. Most children can be treated at home with oral medication, usually by giving an elixir rather than tablets. If hospitalisation is necessary it normally indicates a severe infection and medication may be given by intramuscular injection for the first two days.

211. **B** Penicillin V elixir 125 mg in 5 ml given 6-hourly is a suitable dosage for a 5-year-old child.

212. **C** 5 days is the absolute minimum length of time for a course of penicillin. More than 10 days is rarely required.

213. **A** Children with sore throats are reluctant to eat, but can easily afford to miss food for 2–3 days. Fluids, however, are vital as children may become dehydrated very quickly. Fluids are also important in facilitating the excretion of toxins by the kidneys. Children often have difficulty in gargling and salt water may cause vomiting.

214. **D** Gastro-enteritis (A), colitis (B) and regional ileitis (C – Crohn's disease) are caused by specific infection or inflammatory reaction of the intestine. Mesenteric adenitis refers to inflammation of the lymph glands contained within the mesentery and is quite often a feature of recurrent throat infection.

215. **C**   Loss of appetite is called anorexia. Aphagia (A) means inability to swallow. Anosmia (B) refers to loss of the sense of smell which often results in anorexia. Anabolism (D) refers to the synthesis or building up of tissue by substances derived from digested foods.

216. **B**   An offensive breath is called halitosis. Gingivitis (A) is inflammation of the gums. Hidrosis (C) is the secretion of sweat. Stomatitis (D) is inflammation of the mouth.

217. **B**   Enlarged tonsils are not always indicative of infection. Physiological hypertrophy (enlargement) of the tonsils occurs at about the age of 5 years. After this, in the absence of infection, the tonsils shrink a little but they enlarge again at about the age of 10 years. The school child who is exposed to infection from other children often has enlarged tonsils. Size is therefore of no major significance unless it is considered that they are causing an obstruction.

218. **A**   Most children over the age of 4 years will sit by themselves provided their mother is close by. Over-restraining the child only causes them to be frightened and fractious, thus making the examination very difficult.

219. **C**   Quinsy and peritonsillar abscess are terms used to describe acute inflammation of the tonsil and surrounding tissue, with abscess formation. Follicular tonsillitis (A) describes the situation when the tonsillar crypts are infected and show a white or yellow exudate. Infectious mononucleosis (B) is the correct name for glandular fever in which a sore throat also occurs. Coryza (D) is the correct name for the common cold.

220. **D**   Oedema and infection of the peritonsillar space spreads to the adjacent muscles which are involved when the patient wishes to open the mouth. All of the other symptoms do occur in this disorder but have no specific name.

221. **True**   Most hospitals now issue booklets giving information and simple explanations regarding admission. Many also suggest how best to prepare the child and what to tell him.

222. **True**   If adults tell lies, children lose their confidence and trust in them and become more apprehensive.

223. **False**   Favourite toys are a link with home and serve to comfort the child.

224. **True**   If Christine is actively discouraged from talking about her admission to hospital it will make her think that it is something which is very unpleasant or frightening.

225. **False** Unless the doctor wants to examine her there is no need to wash or undress her immediately. If this is necessary her mother should be allowed to do it.

226. **True** } If there is any sign or recent history of infection the operation should
     and } be postponed because of the greatly increased risk of post-operative
227. **True** } haemorrhage.

228. **False** If tonsillectomy is performed when poliomyelitis is present in the community the virus may gain access to the exposed nerve sheaths and give rise to the more severe and often fatal form of the disease. Vaccination should therefore be given before tonsillectomy is contemplated.

229. **True** Some children of negro race have a genetic abnormality of the haemoglobin which results in sickle-shaped red blood cells. They may have no symptoms apart from mild anaemia but anaesthesia, hypoxaemia or severe infections may precipitate crises in which increased anaemia or capillary thromboses may occur.

230. **False** There is no need for the parents to leave immediately. Free visiting should be allowed and they should spend as much time with the child as they feel able to.

231. **False** Normal supper should be given. Children who are starved for too long a period are quite likely to become hypoglycaemic.

232. **True** Trimeprazine tartrate provides central nervous system sedation and also has anti-emetic properties. Dosage is based on the weight of the child and on the anesthetist's preference for either a sedated child or one who is actually sleeping when anaesthesia is to be induced.

233. **False** Removal by guillotine carries a higher risk of haemorrhage than the more modern technique of dissection.

234. **B** This position allows for the best drainage of secretions.

235. **B** The pulse rate indicates the state of the cardiovascular system and also provides the base line measurement for future comparison should haemorrhage occur. Restlessness (D) immediately post-operatively usually indicates a return to consciousness. Should it occur later it could indicate hidden haemorrhage.

236. **C** Increasing pallor (A) and tachycardia (D) are both signs of haemorrhage. If bleeding is into the pharynx excessive swallowing (B) will be noted. If haemorrhage occurs, the patient's temperature falls rather than increases. Low grade pyrexia means a temperature slightly higher than normal.

237. **A** The sooner the child begins to drink the better. It is important to prevent dehydration, to maintain oral hygiene and to encourage her to swallow.

238. **C** There is always a risk of reactionary haemorrhage. Recording the pulse hourly will give an early indication of this.

239. **D** It is not usually necessary to resort to the more powerful analgesics following tonsillectomy in children. Chloral hydrate is a hypnotic drug of the barbiturate group and will therefore induce sleep but will not relieve pain.

240. **A** A slight elevation of temperature is quite common and subsides quickly. If it persists it usually indicates infection.

241. **D** The sooner the child eats normal food the better. It eases the stiffness and spasm of pharyngeal muscles and dysphagia is relieved in a much shorter time.

242. **D** Pain may be referred along a branch of the glossopharyngeal nerve which serves the area of the tonsillar bed and the middle ear.

243. **True** There is obviously a risk of infection until the tonsillar bed has healed.

244. **True** No special care is needed but sensible precautions should be taken.

245. **False** A white slough is quite normal and should begin to separate 4–8 days post-operatively. Granulation tissue is then seen and after about 3 weeks the mucous membrane should have returned to normal.

246. **False** Referred pain may persist for a short while and is relieved by paracetamol. Should the child appear to be unwell, hot and flushed with persistent earache, then infection should be suspected.

247. **True** Exposure to cold or winds will predispose to earache and infection.

248. **False** 2 weeks usually allows sufficient time for the child to recover in the absence of complications.

Gastric ulceration

Mr Scott is a 50 year old married man, who works as a sales representative for a firm of medical equipment distributors. He has recently been promoted to a new sales area in the North, and as yet has not been able to find a suitable house for his wife and teenage sons.

On returning home one week-end he remarked to his wife that the bouts of indigestion, from which he has been suffering for some time are becoming more frequent. Throughout the week-end he repeatedly complained to his wife of abdominal pain and nausea and on Monday morning she persuaded him to consult his general practitioner.

On consultation the symptoms described by Mr Scott suggested to the general practitioner that he was suffering from a peptic ulcer. To help him confirm his diagnosis the doctor asked Mr Scott a number of questions.

The following questions (249–256) are of the true/false type and consist of a number of statements, some of which are true and some of which are false. Consider each statement and decide whether you think it is true or false. The answers to these questions may be found on pages 46 to 53.

In particular the doctor wished to know if Mr Scott:
249. sleeps well
250. drinks coffee
251. drinks alcohol on an empty stomach
252. rushes his meals
253. avoids fatty food
254. has acid regurgitation
255. has gained weight
256. develops pain after eating spicy food.

249.
250.
251.
252.
253.
254.
255.
256.

Peptic ulceration may occur in either the stomach (gastric ulcer) or in the duodenum (duodenal ulcer). The symptoms of the two are similar but it is unusual for one patient to have both types at the same time. There are however certain distinctive features of each type and these help in determining the diagnosis.

The following questions (257–266) are all of the multiple choice type. Read the questions and from the possible answers select the ONE which you think is correct.

257. Which *one* of the following groups is most likely to exhibit symptoms of gastric ulcer?
    A. Children
    B. Pregnant women
    C. Women in their thirties
    D. Men in their fifties.

257.

258. Which *one* of the following conditions is *not* directly related to the formation of gastric ulcer?
    A. Achlorhydria
    B. Alcoholism
    C. High aspirin intake
    D. Prolonged emotional upset.

258.

259. Which *one* of the following groups of people is most likely to have a high incidence of gastric ulcer?
    A. Non-smokers
    B. People with blood group A
    C. Professional people
    D. Relatives of known ulcer sufferers.

259.

260. Which *one* of the following is a classical description of the pain caused by a gastric ulcer? It occurs:
    A. anytime after eating, but is never relieved by food
    B. an hour after eating and may be relieved by vomiting or food
    C. immediately after eating and is only relieved by vomiting
    D. two hours after eating and is never relieved by food.

260.

Mr Scott told the doctor that he had attempted to relieve the pain with drugs bought from the chemist.

---

261. Which *one* of the following preparations would he be most likely to buy to relieve his symptoms?
    A. Paracetamol
    B. Pro-banthine
    C. Magnesium trisilicate
    D. Duogastrone.

261.

262. Which *one* of the following drugs is *not* an ulcerogenic?
    A. Phenylbutazone
    B. Cortisone
    C. Salicylic acid
    D. Salbutamol.

262.

Mr Scott's general practitioner diagnosed peptic ulceration, and gave him some general advice. Arrangements were made for him to be investigated at the local hospital.

---

263. Which *one* of the following is the most appropriate advice to give to Mr Scott?
    A. Eat normal meals slowly
    B. Eat a bland diet slowly
    C. Eat what you like when you like
    D. Eat only when you are hungry.

263.

264. Which *one* of the following is it *most* important to emphasise to Mr Scott?
    A. Avoid all alcohol
    B. Have only moderate amounts of alcohol
    C. Drink alcohol only if necessary
    D. Avoid taking alcohol on an empty stomach.

264.

265. Which *one* of the following investigations will *not* help in confirmation of the diagnosis?
    A. Barium enema
    B. Barium meal
    C. Gastric secretion test
    D. Fibre optic endoscopy.

265.

266. A number of other tests were also carried out. Which *one* of the following is | 266.
    least likely to have been performed?
    A. Faeces for occult blood
    B. Full blood count
    C. Haemoglobin estimation
    D. Cytology of gastric washings.

There are a number of complications to be considered when caring for a patient with gastric ulcer. The following questions (267–271) consist of a lettered list of groups of symptoms and a numbered list of complications. From the lettered list select *one* group of symptoms for each numbered complication.

267–271 A. Anaemia and slight jaundice   267. Penetration | 267.
         B. Severe pain in the back   268. Malignancy | 268.
         C. Abdominal rigidity, pain and   269. Perforation | 269.
            shock.
         D. Abdominal pain and nausea with   270. Haemorrhage | 270.
            dehydration
         E. Tachycardia, sighing respirations   271. Pyloric stenosis | 271.
            and melaena.

The following questions (272–278) are again of the multiple choice type.

272. Which *one* of the following is *not* a complication of gastric ulceration? | 272.
    A. Perforation
    B. Pyloric stenosis
    C. Haemorrhage
    D. Malignant change.

The doctor suspects that the ulcer is gastric rather than duodenal. Mr Scott is informed that to help confirm this diagnosis an upper gastro-intestinal endoscopy is to be performed. The procedure is explained and he is asked to sign a consent form. He is told that the investigation will be carried out in the Out-patient Department and only a local anaesthetic to the throat and a sedative will be required.)

273. Which *one* of the following *most* accurately describes the area visible during this examination?
   A. Oesophagus
   B. Oesophagus and stomach
   C. Stomach
   D. Oesophagus, stomach and proximal duodenum.

273.

274. Which one of the following is the *most* important part of the investigation in view of Mr Scott's provisional diagnosis?
   A. Photography of any lesions
   B. Noting the number and sites of any ulcers present
   C. Biopsy of all the ulcers present
   D. Noting the number and sites of any ulcers and obtaining cytology specimens.

274.

The results of Mr Scott's investigations showed one gastric ulcer on the lesser curvature of the stomach and no evidence of malignancy. He was advised to continue with his bland diet. Specific drug therapy was commenced.

---

275. Which *one* of the following groups of drugs is thought to promote healing of gastric ulcer?
   A. Antacids
   B. Histamine H_2-receptor antagonists
   C. Anti-emetics
   D. Anticholinergics.

275.

276. Which *one* of the following histamine H_2-receptor antagonists is in common use today?
   A. Mepyramine
   B. Chlorpheniramine
   C. Cimetidine
   D. Metiamide.

276.

277. Cimetidine should be administered:
   A. before breakfast
   B. after main meals
   C. before the evening meal
   D. after lunch.

277.

278. Which *one* of the following is an alternative drug given to promote healing of a gastric ulcer?
     A. Duogastrone
     B. Colloidal bismuth
     C. Biogastrone
     D. Spironolactone.

278.

Mr Scott attended out-patients regularly where his progress was monitored. He did not suffer from any severe haematemesis and no perforation occurred. Either of these would have been an emergency requiring immediate surgery. However after six weeks his ulcer showed no signs of healing and his consultant decided that surgical intervention was now necessary.

The following diagrams (279–282) illustrate different operations for peptic ulcer. Select from the list the correct names for each operation illustrated.

279–282 Operations for peptic ulcer
      A. Polyapartial gastrectomy
      B. Vagotomy and pyloroplasty
      C. Vagotomy and antrectomy
      D. Bilroth I gastrectomy
      E. Truncal vagotomy with drainage

279.
280.
281.
282.

279.

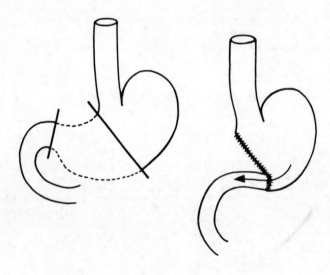

280.

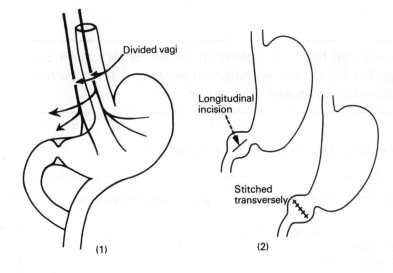

281.

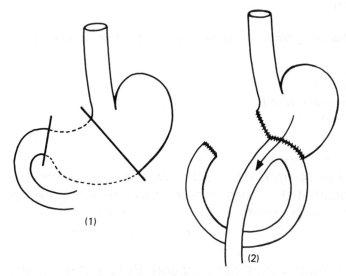

282.

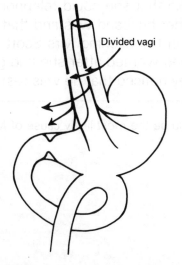

The surgeon decided that the best operation for Mr Scott was a Bilroth I gastrectomy. Mr Scott was admitted to hospital 3 days before his operation to allow for adequate preparation.

The following questions (283–285) are again of the multiple choice type.

283. Which *one* of the following is *not* essential as part of his pre-operative preparation?
   A. High protein diet with added vitamins
   B. Correction of anaemia
   C. Deep breathing exercises
   D. Stomach washout

283.

284. Which *one* of the following blood investigations would *not* be necessary pre-operatively?
   A. Full blood count
   B. Prothrombin estimation
   C. Group and cross match blood
   D. Haemoglobin estimation.

284.

On the day before the operation Mr Scott was seen by both the surgeon and the anaesthetist. It was explained to him what the operation entailed and arrangements were made for him to have a sedative should he require it. Mr Scott seemed quite satisfied and glad that something was being done at last.

In the evening Mrs Scott visited her husband. Before she left she spoke to the sister. She was told that she could telephone the ward the next afternoon to ask how her husband was and that she should be able to visit him for a while in the evening Mrs Scott was unduly agitated and her husband seemed worried after she had gone. When the night staff came on duty they noticed that he was restless.

285. Which *one* of the following would be the *most* likely cause of Mr Scott's anxiety after his wife's visit?
   A. Fear of the operation
   B. Fear of the anaesthetic
   C. Problems at home
   D. Fear of losing his job.

285.

On the morning of the operation Mr Scott was taken to theatre.

The following questions are all of the true/false type (286–292).

It is the responsibility of the nurse in charge to check:

286. his name and record number with the case notes   286.

287. any allergy to drugs   287.

288. that the pre-medication has been given   288.

289. all relevant X-rays are present   289.

290. the abdomen has been shaved   290.

291. that he has passed urine   291.

292. that a telephone number is available for contacting his relatives 292.

Following the operation a qualified nurse went from the ward to theatre to collect Mr Scott. Before leaving theatre she should obtain certain items of information from the anaesthetist.

The following questions (293–308) are all of the multiple choice type.

293. Which *one* of the following facts is it *not* immediately essential for her to know?
  A. The exact operation performed
  B. The type of anaesthetic given
  C. The intravenous fluid regime
  D. The general condition of the patient.

293.

294. Whilst Mr Scott is unconscious his airway must be maintained. In order to do this he must be nursed in which *one* of the following positions?
  A. Recumbent
  B. Semiprone
  C. Prone
  D. Semi-recumbent.

294.

295. In which *one* of the following positions should Mr Scott be nursed once he has regained consciousness?
  A. Sim's
  B. Prone
  C. Semi-recumbent
  D. Lithotomy.

295.

296. On his return from theatre a nasogastric (Ryle's) tube will be in situ. This should be aspirated:
  A. continuously
  B. when necessary, as the patient demands
  C. every two to four hours
  D. hourly and when there is nausea.

296.

297. Before *each* aspiration of the gastric contents the nurse should:
  A. insert 20 mls of water to ensure patency
  B. aspirate, and check the pH of the aspirate
  C. move the Ryle's tube up and down
  D. place the end of the tube under water.

297.

298. A nasogastric tube is usually inserted to:
    A. reduce pain and vomiting
    B. allow gastric feeding
    C. facilitate gastric analysis
    D. prevent haematemisis.

298.

299. The fluid of choice for intravenous infusion is *most* likely to be:
    A. 5% Dextrose
    B. Hartmann's Solution
    C. Dextrose 4.3%. Saline 0.18%
    D. Darrow's Solution.

299.

The doctor will discontinue Mr Scott's infusion when his bowel sounds return and he can tolerate fluids by mouth. While the infusion is in progress the nurse must watch the patient carefully and report any abnormal findings.

---

300. Which *one* of the following is the responsibility of the doctor rather than the nurse?
    A. Monitor and regulate the rate of flow
    B. Decrease the rate of infusion as Mr Scott's condition improves
    C. Record the amount of fluid infused accurately
    D. Observe the cannula site for inflammation and oedema.

300.

301. When Mr Scott recovers consciousness, which *one* of the following should the nurse do first?
    A. Give him a mouthwash
    B. Reassure him
    C. Tell him his wife has telephoned
    D. Give him extra pillows.

301.

To ensure Mr Scott's comfort and co-operation analgesia will be prescribed to be given four to six hourly for 48 hours.

---

302. The *most* likely post-operative analgesia would be:
    A. dihydrocodeine 50 mg
    B. hyoscine 0.4 mg
    C. trimeprazine 10 mg
    D. pethidine 50 mg.

302.

303. To minimise post-operative complications, mobilisation should begin: 303.
    A. within six hours
    B. after twenty-four hours
    C. within twenty-four hours
    D. within three days.

As soon as Mr Scott returns to the ward from theatre the nurse should check the wound site(s). Thereafter the wound and the dressing will need to be checked at regular intervals throughout the post-operative period.

304. Which *one* of the following is the *least* important point for the nurse to note   304.
    when checking the wound?
    A. Number of wound drains inserted
    B. Number of sutures inserted
    C. Type of wound drains inserted
    D. Type of sutures inserted.

When the nurse checks the wound it is important that she should note and report any signs which might indicate infection.

305. Which *one* of the following is *not* necessarily a sign of infection?   305.
    A. Swelling
    B. Discolouration
    C. Offensive odour
    D. Heat and redness.

306. Which *one* of the following statements is most accurate? Wound drains   306.
    should be removed:
    A. by the third day
    B. when drainage ceases
    C. after they have been shortened once
    D. only when an analgesic has been given.

Mr Scott had an uneventful recovery and by the tenth post-operative day he was ready for discharge. His wife had been kept fully informed of his progress and was pleased to be having him home.

307. Which *one* of the following statements is the best advice to give to Mr Scott regarding his meals?
    A. Eat normal-sized meals
    B. Drink plenty of fluid with meals
    C. Continue with his bland diet
    D. Lie down after meals if he feels faint.

307.

308. Which *one* of the following statements is true regarding Mr Scott's return to work and his future health?
    A. He should be back at work within a month
    B. He should avoid heavy lifting for at least eight weeks
    C. Further Out-Patient appointments will not be necessary
    D. Further gastric surgery will not be necessary.

308.

Gastric ulceration answers and explanations

249. **True**   Nocturnal pain is a common symptom of peptic ulceration.

250. **False**   This would be appropriate only if the patient drank strong coffee continually on an empty stomach.

251. **True**   Alcohol is also an irritant. It is often a contributory factor in peptic ulcer.

252. **True**   Ulcers are often associated with rushed meals. Because of his type of work Mr Scott frequently finds it convenient to have a quick pub lunch.

253. **True**   Fried food may cause an exacerbation of the dyspepsia.

254. **True**   This may occur if there is excessive acid in the stomach.

255. **False**   In peptic ulcer there is more likely to be weight loss.

256. **True**   Spicy food predisposes to dyspepsia.

257. **D**   Gastric and duodenal ulcer are both rare in children (A). The incidence is lower in women than in men and the symptoms are rarely seen in pregnancy (B). The average age of onset for gastric ulcer in men is 50–59 years. In women (C) the onset is later – usually in their sixties. In duodenal ulcer the age of onset is usually 40–49 years in women and 30–39 years in men.

258. **A**   Reasons for ulcer formation are not yet fully understood but they never occur in the absence of hydrochloric acid (A). (B), (C) and (D) may all be predisposing factors.

259. **D**   Gastric ulcer seems to be more common in people with a family history of the condition. People in the other three groups have not been shown to have a significantly high incidence of gastric ulcer. For some unknown reason people with blood group A, B and AB are less likely to develop gastric ulcer than those with group O blood (B). It also occurs more commonly in the lower social classes than in professional people (C). Smoking (A) is an irritant but it has not been shown actually to cause ulceration, although it may exacerbate the condition where it already exists.

260. **B** This is the classical description of the pain cycle caused by a gastric ulcer. In fact a duodenal ulcer may show the same manifestations. The pain occurs more quickly after food in gastric ulcer but in both the pain is relieved by eating.

261. **C** Magnesium trisilicate is the only safe drug which he could buy over the counter. Pro-banthine (B) and Duogastrone (D) are only available on prescription. Paracetamol (A) is a mild analgesic but it would not relieve his gastric symptoms.

262. **D** Ulcerogenic means ulcer-causing. This is a side effect of all the drugs listed except salbutamol (which is a broncho-dilator). For this reason (A), (B) and (C) are best avoided by people suffering from gastric ulcer.

263. **B** It is important that Mr Scott eats his meals slowly, in a relaxed atmosphere and at regular intervals. He should avoid highly spiced food.

264. **D** Mr Scott need not give up alcohol altogether. However, alcohol is an irritant so if food is taken before drinking it will act as a 'buffer' and help to prevent dyspepsia.

265. **A** Mr Scott's symptoms indicate that the cause lies higher up the digestive tract than would be demonstrated by barium enema. The other tests listed could all help with confirmation of the diagnosis. The barium meal (B) would show irregularities in the oesophagus, stomach and duodenum. These would also be seen by fibre optic endoscopy (D). In addition this technique permits photography of the stomach and cytology specimens to be taken. The gastric secretion test (C) will allow the level of acid in the stomach to be estimated. Patients with ulcers tend to have hyperchlorhydria. Those with pernicious anaemia or gastric carcinoma tend to have achlorhydria.

266. **D** Cytology of gastric washings is rarely undertaken today. There may be an eroded blood vessel causing chronic bleeding. This blood is not visible to the naked eye but can be detected by chemical means (occult blood test) (A). The obvious presence of altered blood in the faeces, when the stools are distinctively black and tarry, is called melaena.
A full blood count (B) and haemoglobin estimation (C) are methods of detecting anaemia which may have resulted from chronic bleeding.

267. **B** Penetration of an ulcer will give rise to severe pain in the back and exacerbation of other symptoms.

268. **A** The early signs of malignancy are anaemia and slight jaundice with unexpected weight loss.

269. **C** A patient with a perforated ulcer presents with sudden, severe abdominal pain and shock. The abdomen is rigid and the breathing is shallow. Bowel sounds are absent. The onset is sudden and frequently follows a meal.

270. **E** If the ulcer erodes a major blood vessel severe haemorrhage will occur and the patient will show all the signs of hypovolaemic shock. There will be melaena and/or haematemesis.

271. **D** When there is scar tissue around the pyloric sphincter the passage of food from the stomach is obstructed. This causes pain, nausea and dehydration leading to malnutrition and weight loss.

272. **B** Pyloric stenosis is more commonly a complication of duodenal ulcer. The other complications listed may all occur in gastric ulcer. Haemorrhage (C) may be acute when a major blood vessel is eroded. This will result in haematemesis and melaena. Chronic haemorrhage may be hidden but can be demonstrated by a positive result from stools tested for occult blood. Perforation (A) may also occur and is the commonest cause of death. There is severe pain with the escape of gastric contents into the peritoneal cavity causing irritation of the peritoneum and the development of general peritonitis within 12 hours. Malignant changes (D) occur in approximately 6 per cent of patients with gastric ulcer.

273. **D** After passing the fibreoptic endoscope, the interior of the oesophagus, stomach and proximal duodenum can be seen. Colour or cine photographs may be taken during this procedure. A tissue biopsy for cytological examination may also be obtained.

274. **D** This would probably be the most comprehensive plan for the examination. Sometimes only photographs (A) or only biopsies of the ulcers (C) may be taken, but as Mr Scott's symptoms have been present for some time the cytology may be significant.

275. **B** Histamine H_2 – receptor antagonists inhibit the secretion of gastric acid and thus potentiate ulcer healing. Anticholinergic drugs (D) inhibit parasympathetic activity and reduce gastric motility. They are useful in the relief of continuous pain, especially at night, as they allow anatacids to remain in the stomach longer. Antacids (A) are substances which neutralise acidity. Anti-emetics (C) prevent vomiting.

276. **C** Cimetidine (Tagamet) is the drug in question. It reduces both resting and stimulated gastric acid production. Metiamide (D) was an early H_2 – receptor antagonist which was withdrawn when cimetidine was developed. Mepyramine (A) is an antihistamine useful in the treatment of allergic skin conditions. Chlorpheniramine (B) is a short-acting antihistamine.

277. **B** This drug should be given orally, three times daily after meals. This will slow the rate of absorption of the drug and allow peak blood levels to be achieved, even when the stomach is empty.

278. **C** Biogastrone (carbenoxolone) is sodium derived from liquorice root. It increases mucosal resistance but does not affect gastric acid production and is ineffective for duodenal ulcers.
Duogastrone (A) is carbenoxolone is a gelatine capsule which is formulated for release in the duodenum.
Spironolactone (Aldactone) is a diuretic. Colloidal bismuth (B) will promote healing but its effect on ulcer recurrence is unknown at present.

279. **D** Bilroth I Gastrectomy – a partial gastrectomy with a duodenal anastomosis.

280. **B** Vagotomy and pyloroplasty.

281. **A** Polypartial gastrectomy

282. **E** Truncal vagotomy with drainage.

283. **D** A stomach washout is not an essential part of the pre-operative preparation. Although the stomach must be empty this can be achieved by fasting. Withhholding food and fluid for 4–6 hours pre-operatively is usually sufficient but in preparation for gastric surgery most anaethesists prefer a longer period of fasting, usually about 12 hours. This reduces the risk of vomiting and acid regurgitation.
A high protein diet with added vitamins (A) is necessary to promote healthy tissue and to ensure successful healing.
Anaemia (B) should be corrected since a correct level of haemoglobin will ensure adequate tissue oxygenation.
Deep breathing exercises (C) are important to help clear the chest of secretions pre- and post-operatively, especially if the patient smokes.

284. **B** Normally there would be no reason to estimate prothrombin levels. Estimations of haemoglobin (D) and a full blood count (A) would both be required to give a base-line for post-operative assessment. Grouping and cross-matching of 2–3 units of blood (C) is carried out, and this blood is given by transfusion during or after the operation to replace blood lost and to counteract shock.

285. **C** Worry about affairs at home is likely to be the main cause of his anxiety. The nurse should be aware of this and if necessary arrangements should be made for him to talk to the medical social worker as soon as possible. The medical social worker will provide help and advice regarding any problems related to finance or employment. Since Mr Scott is in regular work and has recently been promoted he is unlikely to lose his job (D) as a result of a period of sick leave.
Any fears relating to the operation (A) or the anaesthetic (B) should have been allayed already by the surgeon and the anaesthetist.

286. **True** It is most important to check that the correct notes have gone with the patient or he may receive the wrong operation.

287. **False** This should have already been done by medical staff.

288. **True**

289. **True**

290. **True**

291. **True** He should at least have had the opportunity to do so.

292. **False** This would have already been checked on admission and should be in his notes.

293. **B** The nurse should be told if oxygen has had to be given in the recovery room but it is not necessary for her to have details of drugs given for anaethesia at this stage as they will be written up in the operation notes. It is essential that she receives verbal and written reports on his general condition (D), the operation carried out (A) and the planned intravenous fluid regime (C).

294. **B** Nursing the patient semi-prone, on either side, positioned with pillows, allows a free airway and drainage of secretions from the mouth and nose (see Figure).

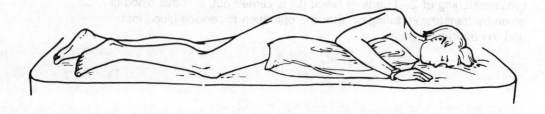

295. **C** On recovering consciousness he may be nursed flat with one pillow, on his back or either side. Within 12 hours he should be sitting up, comfortably supported by pillows. This allows for better lung expansion.

296. **D** The Ryle's tube is usually aspirated hourly or if the patient feels sick. But sometimes it may be necessary to allow continuous free drainage. Occasionally a Robert's pump may be used. The time lapse between aspirations will be extended if the doctor requests it.

297. **B** The pH of the aspirate should be checked each time to ensure that the tube is still in the stomach. It is only necessary to check the patency of the tube (A) or to move it (C) if it appears to be blocked. Placing the end of the tube under water (D) is an additional check that the tube is not in the lungs and might be done when it is inserted.

298. **A** By regularly removing gastric contents and gas the pressure on the internal sutures is reduced and there is therefore less pain. As the stomach remains fairly empty there is also less likelihood of vomiting. Gastric feeding (B) is inappropriate as oral feeding will commence quite soon. Gastric analysis (C) is carried out preoperatively. A nasogastric tube will not prevent haematemesis (D).

299. **C** Dextrose 4.3 per cent and saline 0.18 per cent will provide sodium and chloride as well as water and carbohydrates. This solution will therefore replace fluid and electrolyte loss during surgery and will also provide calories while the patient is unable to take food by mouth. 5 per cent dextrose (A) provides calories and water but no electrolytes. Hartmann's solution (B) is useful to correct acidosis. It provides electrolytes and water but no calories. Darrow's solution (D) is used for the correction of extracellular fluid depletion with mild potassium loss and acidosis. It is unlikely to be used in this case.

300. **B** The rate of infusion must be decided by the doctor. It is not the responsibility of the nurse. She should accurately monitor and regulate the rate of flow (A) in accordance with the doctor's instructions and should maintain an accurate fluid chart (C). Inflammation or oedema at the cannula site (D) must be reported as these are signs of infection or escape of fluid into the tissues.

301. **B** Before she does anything else the nurse should speak to him quietly and reassure him that all is well.

302. **D** Pethidine is the analgesic of choice as it has minimal side effects and is less likely to cause respiratory depression than dihydrocodeine (A). Hyoscine (B) and trimeprazine (C) are used as pre-operative sedatives.

303. **C** Mobilisation should begin as soon as possible but the effects of the anaesthetic are likely to last for up to six hours (A). If the patient's condition is poor, mobilisation will be delayed (B and D).

304. **B** The number of sutures inserted is relatively unimportant. However the type of suture used (D) is important to note as this may influence the day of removal. For example clips are removed after 5–6 days, interrupted sutures will usually be left in for 8–9 days, while continuous sutures are not taken out until the 10th day. If the wound becomes infected it may be necessary to remove some of the sutures earlier. The number (A) and type (C) of wound drains used is also important to note as this will influence the post-operative management. For example a vacuum suction drain will need to have the vacuum renewed 4-hourly and will be removed by the 3rd day. A corrugated drain may need frequent dressing and will normally be shortened after 24 hours and removed after 48 hours.
Correct management of both sutures and drains is important as they both present potential sites for infection and delayed wound healing.

305. **B** Some operations involve a considerable amount of local trauma which may result in post-operative bruising but on its own this is not a sign of infection.

306. **B** This is the best guide to the time for removal. Some may be removed after 48 hours but some will be left in situ for longer (A). Not all drains require shortening (C).
An analgesic (D) should not be needed unless the patient is very anxious.

307. **D** Sometimes after a partial gastrectomy patients complain of a feeling of fullness, nausea, giddiness and extreme fatigue occurring during a meal or immediately afterwards when the patient is in the upright position. This is known as the 'dumping syndrome'. It is thought to be due to jejunal distension and vasodilation of the intestinal wall creating a drop in circulating plasma volume. The patient may also complain of tachcardia and sweating. The symptoms are relieved by lying down after meals. The condition can be avoided by eating small meals (A) at frequent intervals and by not drinking at the same time (B).
Following partial gastrectomy it is not normally necessary to continue with a bland diet (C) although highly spiced foods and very hot fluids should still be avoided.

308. **B** Following any major abdominal surgery heavy lifting should be avoided to reduce the risk of incisional hernia. As Mr Scott's work involved a lot of travelling and irregular hours he will need to convalesce for at least three months (A). A number of late post-operative complications may develop, such as anaemia, and for this reason Mr Scott must continue to attend out-patients regularly as requested (C). If the dumping syndrome persists he may require further surgery (D).

Cholecystectomy

Miss Jean Flynn, aged 48 years, is a primary school teacher who lives alone in a block of flats. She enjoys cooking and often entertains her friends. Her mother, aged 70, is still very active and visits Jean regularly. During her visits her main topic of conversation is her daughter's incessant smoking and her need to lose weight.

For some months Jean has suffered from attacks of upper abdominal pain and nausea. This has caused her increasing absences from work and it has now been thought necessary to admit her to hospital for investigation.

After taking her history the doctor made a provisional diagnosis of cholecystitis.

The following questions (309–323) are all of the multiple choice type. Read the questions and from the possible answers select the ONE which you think is correct. You can indicate your answer by writing the appropriate letter in the right hand margin. The answers to these questions may be found on pages 62–67.

309. Acute cholecystitis most commonly occurs in:
    A. obese men in their fifties
    B. obese women in their forties
    C. young pregnant women
    D. men and women over 60.

309.

310. The organism most commonly associated with acute infection of the gall bladder is:
    A. Streptococcus faecalis
    B. Staphylococcus aureus
    C. Escherichia coli
    D. Streptococcus viridans.

310.

311. Acute cholecystitis:
    A. always occurs with primary infection
    B. is never present without obstruction
    C. is frequently due to cholelithiasis
    D. frequently results from a staphylococcal infection.

311.

312. Obstruction commonly occurs in the:
    A. right hepatic duct
    B. cystic duct
    C. sphincter of Oddi
    D. gall bladder.

312.

313. Obstructive acute cholecystitis causes pain in the: 313.
    A. left hypochondrium
    B. left lumbar region
    C. hypogastrium
    D. right hypochondrium.

314. Patients with cholecystitis should be advised to: 314.
    A. avoid all fat
    B. have a low fat diet
    C. take plenty of carbohydrate
    D. take regular aperients.

When the doctor examined Jean he noticed that she was slightly jaundiced. Her temperature was raised and she complained of nausea and occasional vomiting in addition to her abdominal pain.

---

315. Jaundice indicates obstruction of which *one* of the following ducts?   315.
    A. Left hepatic
    B. Cystic
    C. Common bile
    D. Pancreatic.

316. Which *one* of the following groups are *all* symptoms of obstructive jaundice?   316.
    A. Fatty stools, yellow skin, pale urine
    B. Pale stools, dark urine, raised serum urobilinogen
    C. Yellow sclera, offensive stools, low serum urobilinogen
    D. Itchy skin, yellow sclera, dark stools.

317. Which *one* of the following investigations is undertaken to demonstrate   317.
    stones in the gall bladder?
    A. Cholangiogram
    B. Cystogram
    C. Cystometrogram
    D. Cholecystogram.

318. Which *one* of the following is undertaken to demonstrate stones in the   318.
    common bile duct?
    A. Cholangiogram
    B. Cystogram
    C. Cystometrogram
    D. Cholecystogram.

The doctor decided to send Jean for a cholecystogram. For this investigation the patient is asked to swallow a compound containing radio-opaque iodine. In preparation for this Jean was given a low residue diet for 24 hours and then fasted for 10 hours immediately prior to the X-ray. She was also given an iodine sensitivity test which was found to be negative.

319. A cholecystogram will demonstrate the gall bladder in all but *one* of the following conditions. Which one?
    A. The left hepatic duct is obstructed
    B. The sphincter of Oddi is obstructed
    C. The cystic duct is blocked
    D. Cholecystokinin secretion is impaired.

319.

Jean's cholecystogram failed to demonstrate the gall bladder and the doctor therefore decided to send her for a cholangiogram. Since she had already been tested for sensitivity to iodine no special preparation was required.

320. In a cholangiogram radioactive iodine is given:
    A. intramuscularly
    B. intravenously
    C. orally
    D. rectally.

320.

The cholangiogram demonstrated the presence of stones in the gall bladder and biliary tract.

When Jean was settled for the night she was given a mild analgesic but 2 hours later she complained to the night nurse of a sudden severe colicky pain and she was very restless. The nurse also noted that her temperature was slightly raised and her pulse rate was rapid.

321. Jean's sudden pain and restlessness is most likely to indicate:
    A. peritonitis
    B. perforation of the gall bladder
    C. obstruction of the common biliary duct
    D. an allergic reaction to the intravenous iodine.

321.

322. The doctor is *most* likely to prescribe morphine sulphate 15–20 mg for Jean's pain because it is:
    A. a strong analgesic
    B. an effective antispasmodic
    C. able to promote peristalsis
    D. a muscle relaxant.

322.

323. The doctor also prescribed propantheline bromide 30 mg. This was given to:
    A. increase gastric secretions
    B. relieve spasm
    C. increase biliary secretion
    D. relieve anxiety.

323.

Next morning the surgeon decided that it was time to operate. He told Jean that he intended to remove her gall bladder and examine her common bile duct.

324–327. The following questions are all matching items. From the list on the left select the statement which describes each operation listed on the right.

A. Removal of the gall bladder	324. Cholecystostomy	324.
B. Drainage of the common bile duct	325. Cholecystectomy	325.
C. Removal of stones from the common bile duct	326. Choledochostomy	326.
D. Drainage of the gall bladder	327. Choledocholithotomy	327.

The doctor came and took a sample of blood as part of Jean's pre-operative preparation.

The following questions (328–344) are once again of the multiple choice type.

---

328. Which *one* of the following blood examinations would *not* be necessary?
    A. Grouping
    B. Prothrombin time
    C. Haemoglobin
    D. White cell count.

328.

329. Patients with obstructive jaundice are likely to suffer from deficiency of which *one* of the following vitamins?
    A. A
    B. D
    C. E
    D. K.

329.

330. Women with obstructive jaundice have an increased risk of bleeding because:
    A. their prothrombin level is high
    B. they are unable to digest fat
    C. they are usually overweight
    D. they are usually of childbearing age.

330.

331. Which *one* of the following groups of factors is involved in the bloodclotting mechanism?
    A. Platelets, vitamin E and prothrombin
    B. Prothrombin, vitamin K and calcium
    C. Thromboplastin, vitamin A and iron
    D. Fibrinogen, vitamin K and sodium citrate.

331.

332. Patients who have obstructive jaundice may be given:
    A. cyanocobalamin
    B. phytomenadione
    C. riboflavin
    D. thiamine.

332.

Jean's blood investigations were satisfactory and she was prepared for surgery. After being given a pre-medication she was transferred to theatre, where the operation was carried out as planned.

333. On return to the ward which *one* of the following should have priority?
    A. The administration of an analgesic
    B. Unclamping and commencing drainage of the T tube
    C. Giving breathing exercises
    D. Reading the operation notes.

333.

334. An intravenous infusion of Dextrose 4.3% and Saline 0.18% had been set up in theatre. The surgeon gave instructions to continue with 500 mls every four hours. At this rate of flow the number of drops per minute (to the nearest whole number) is:
    A. 15
    B. 23
    C. 31
    D. 47

334.

335. The intravenous infusion will probably be discontinued:
    A. after 24 hours
    B. when oral fluids are tolerated
    C. after 48 hours
    D. when oral fluids are tolerated and peristalsis is present.

335.

Jean also had a nasogastric tube *in situ*. This was aspirated hourly at first.

336. When aspirating the nasogastic tube the nurse should:
      A. increase the time between aspirations
      B. offer oral fluids hourly
      C. instil clear fluid after each aspiration
      D. offer mouth washes frequently.

336.

337. During the first 12 hours following operation the nurse was instructed to:
      A. commence oral fluids
      B. get Jean out of bed
      C. make regular observations of pulse and blood pressure
      D. inspect the wound 4-hourly.

337.

338. Jean has two tubes coming from her operation site. One of these is a T-tube which drains:
      A. the gall bladder bed
      B. the duodenum
      C. the hepatic duct
      D. the common bile duct.

338.

Jean's T-tube will eventually be removed. While it remains in situ certain routine procedures are necessary. The T-tube will be clamped intermittently after 48 hours.

---

339. The T-tube will not be clamped completely until:
      A. the fifth day
      B. the eighth day
      C. after 24 hours of intermittent clamping
      D. after intermittent clamping occurs without pain.

339.

340. Before the T-tube is removed it should remain clamped for:
      A. 6 hours
      B. 12 hours
      C. 18 hours
      D. 24 hours.

340.

341. Which one of the following indicates obstruction to the flow of bile when the T-tube is clamped?
      A. Absence of bile in the urine
      B. Stools contain bile pigments
      C. Biliary colic
      D. Diminishing biliary drainage.

341.

342. Which *one* of the following investigations will be carried out to check patency of the biliary system, before the T-tube is removed?
    A. Operative cholangiogram
    B. Percutaneous cholangiogram
    C. T-tube cholangiogram
    D. Intravenous cholangiogram.

    342.

343. After the removal of the tube the nurse should observe the fistula daily for signs of:
    A. infection
    B. excess bile drainage
    C. haemorrhage
    D. serous drainage.

    343.

344. The usual time for the removal of sutures is:
    A. 6–8 days
    B. 8–10 days
    C. 10–12 days
    D. 12–14 days.

    344.

Jean made an uneventful recovery. Shortly after the removal of the T-tube and her sutures she was told she could arrange to go home. It was agreed that she should go and stay with her mother for the first few days but she was assured that as soon as she felt well enough she could return to live alone in her own flat. However the Sister advised her that she should arrange to have help with any heavy housework and that she would need to stay off work for at least three or four months.

The doctor told her that she should now be able to resume a normal diet but he advised her to watch her weight and to try to give up smoking.

Before she left the hospital she was given an appointment to attend the out-patients department in 4 weeks' time. After that she planned to go for a restful holiday before returning to work.

Cholecystectomy Answers and explanations

309. **B**   Cholecystitis most commonly occurs in women who are obese and have had many children – 'fair, fat, female, fertile and forty'.

310. **C**   Streptococcus faecalis (A) and streptococcus viridans (D) may be found to be the causal organism but E. coli is the commonest.

311. **C**   Acute cholecystitis usually occurs following obstruction of the bile duct by a gall stone. It rarely occurs as a primary infection without obstruction, although this may occur when the gall bladder is acting as a reservoir for the typhoid bacillus.

312. **B**   The cystic duct is the commonest site of obstruction. Although gall stones are formed in the gall bladder they rarely cause symptoms until they pass into the biliary tract.

313. **D**   In acute cholecystitis the pain is characteristically in the right hypochondrium over the gall bladder.

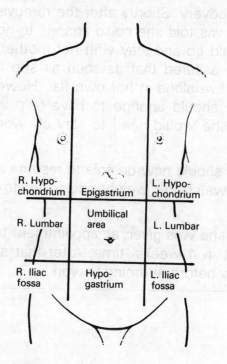

Regions of the abdomen

314. **B** Some fat should be retained in the diet to encourage the gall bladder to empty and so prevent biliary stasis. These patients tend to be overweight and should be encouraged to reduce their carbohydrate intake (C). Aperients should never be taken regularly (D), only as required.

315. **C** Jaundice occurs because the flow of bile from the liver to the duodenum is obstructed. Obstruction of the left hepatic duct (A) will only partially interfere with the flow (see Fig.). Obstruction of the cystic duct (B) will cause stasis of the bile already in the gall bladder, possibly leading to infection.

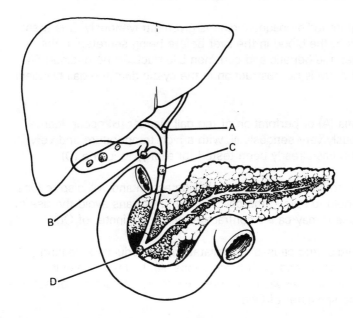

Sites of biliary tract obstruction
A. Hepatic duct
B. Cystic duct
C. Common bile duct
D. Sphincter of Oddi.

316. **B** In obstructive jaundice bile is prevented from entering the duodenum. This results in pale, clay-coloured stools which contain much undigested fat and are very offensive. The liver cannot deal with the excess bile pigments which therefore accumulate in the blood stream causing an itchy yellow skin and yellow sclera. The excess is excreted via the kidneys giving a dark colour to the urine. The serum urobilinogen is high.

317. **D** A cholecystogram demonstrates gall bladder appearance and function.

318. **A** A cholangiogram is undertaken to demonstrate the presence of gall stones or strictures in the hepatic or common bile ducts. Cystograms (D) and cystometrograms (C) are special X-rays of the urinary bladder.

319. **C** Demonstration of the gall bladder in cholecystography depends upon the normal secretion of bile containing the radio-opaque iodine which is then concentrated in the gall bladder. If the production of bile is impaired or if its flow to the gall bladder is obstructed (C) this cannot take place. Cholecystokinin (D) stimulates the gall bladder to contract and if this fails to happen the bile ducts will not be demonstrated on the X-ray.

320. **B** In a cholangiogram radio-opaque iodine is given intravenously. It is then concentrated from the blood in the liver before being secreted in the bile. This enables the hepatic and common bile ducts to be outlined on X-ray. Provided there is no obstruction in the cystic duct the gall bladder will be visible.

321. **C** Should peritonitis (A) or perforation of the gall bladder (B) occur Jean would be obviously very seriously ill, with a high temperature and very rapid pulse. Jean has already been tested for allergy to iodine (D).

322. **A** Morphine sulphate has a strong pain relieving action and will also reduce peristalsis and help to relieve the colic. Some physicians avoid the use of this drug because it may cause contracture at the sphincter of Oddi.

323. **B** This anticholinergic drug causes vasodilatation and reduces sweating, salivation and bronchial and gastric secretions (A). In Jean's case it would be given as an antispasmodic primarily to counteract the effect of morphine on the sphincter of Oddi.

324. **D**

325. **A**

326. **B**

327. **C**

328. **D** The haemoglobin level (C) and blood group (A) are determined before all major operations. In patients with obstructive jaundice it is necessary to estimate the prothrombin time but a white cell count is not essential. The prothrombin time is the time taken for plasma to clot after the addition of thromboplastin. It is a measure of the prothrombin concentration in the blood. The normal time is 11–18 seconds.

329. **D** Vitamin K is absorbed from the intestine in the presence of bile salts. In obstructive jaundice the flow of bile into the duodenum is interrupted, inhibiting the absorption of vitamin K.

330. **B** Any patient with obstructive jaundice is unable to digest fat properly because of the lack of bile entering the duodenum. Bile salts are essential for the breakdown of fat. Vitamin K is a fat soluble vitamin and is essential for the formation of prothrombin.

331. **B** The factors necessary for the clotting of blood are: prothrombin and vitamin K, calcium, platelets and thromboplastin, fibrinogen. (See diagram)
Sodium citrate (D) delays blood clotting. Iron (C) is a constituent of haemoglobin.

Vitamin K + Plasma prothrombin + Calcium + Thromboplastin ◄——Blood platelets

Thrombin + Fibrinogen

Fibrin mesh (clot)

332. **B** Phytomenadione (Konakion) is a preparation of vitamin K. The others all belong to the B group of vitamins.

333. **B** Establishing free drainage is of immediate importance. Analgesia (A) and breathing exercises (C) will be required but not immediately. The operation notes are not likely to have been written up yet by the doctor (D) and in any case the nurse should have ascertained the important details when collecting the patient from theatre.

334. **B** The formula for calculating the rate of flow is:
$$\frac{\text{Number of ml per bottle (bag)}}{\text{Number of hours to be given in}} \times \frac{\text{Number of drops per ml}}{\text{Number of minutes per hour}}$$

There are 15 drops in 1 ml, therefore if a patient is to be given 500 ml of fluid over a 4-hour period, the formula will look like this:

$$\frac{500}{4} \times \frac{15}{60} = \frac{125}{4} = 31.25 \text{ (31 drops)}$$

335. **D** This is a medical decision but the criteria to be taken into consideration are the patient's toleration of oral fluids and the return of peristalsis.

336. **D** The nurse should not alter the time between aspirations (A), offer oral fluids (B) or instil fluid via the tube (C) without medical instruction. Mouthwashes should be offered frequently to relieve the discomfort of a dry mouth.

337. **C** Observations of pulse and blood pressure will be required during the first 24 hours. Oral fluids (A) will not be started unless bowel sounds have returned. The patient will be encouraged to get up and start moving after 24 hours (B). The dressing should be inspected regularly but the wound should not be uncovered unless the dressing needs changing (D).

338. **D** See diagram. B is the T-tube in the common bile duct.
The other drain (A on the diagram) is in the gall bladder bed to prevent the formation of haematoma.

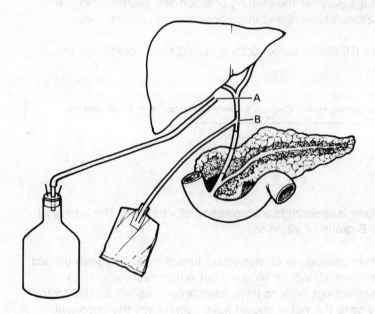

339. **D** Provided the intermittent clamping does not cause pain it will be continued for longer periods each day until there is very little or no bile draining into the collecting bag. When this stage is reached it will be removed.

340. **D** Leaving the tube clamped for 24 hours allows time for any signs of obstruction to be detected.

341. **C** If the flow of bile is obstructed the biliary colic will return. The urine (A) will contain bile but there will be an absence of bile pigments in the stools (B). If the T-tube is clamped it will not be possible to assess the amount of bile drainage (D).

342. **C** A T-tube cholangiogram is carried out approximately 10 days post-operatively in order to confirm the patency of the duct before removing the T-tube.

343. **B** Bile escaping from the wound will cause excoriation of the skin which the nurse must avoid by applying daily dressings if necessary. Daily observations of temperature and pulse will give an earlier indication of infection (A). Post-operative haemorrhage at this stage is unlikely (C).

344. **B** 8–10 days unless the wound is not healed or the surgeon directs otherwise.

Ulcerative colitis

Anne Mitchell, aged 21 years, lives at home with her parents. Her mother is in her late fifties and her father his middle sixties. She has no brothers or sisters. Anne has tended to live a rather sheltered life and has been very over-protected by her parents. Their home is a comfortable villa in the residential area of the city.

Anne is now studying at university for a Master of Arts degree and hopes eventually to become a teacher. Unfortunately she has fallen well behind with her studies due to repeated attacks of acute diarrhoea which have meant absences from the university of several weeks at a time. During one such acute attack she had to be admitted to hospital.

On admission she was rather emotional. Her appearance was that of a pale, thin, anxious, young woman. Observations made by the nurse admitting her to an acute medical ward were recorded and a report was given to the sister. From the history given by herself and her parents a provisional diagnosis of ulcerative colitis was made by the doctor.

The following questions (345–389) are all of the multiple choice type. Read the questions and from the possible answers select the ONE which you think is correct. You can indicate your answer by writing the appropriate letter in the right hand margin. The answers to these questions may be found on pages 79–85.

345. In which *one* of the following groups does ulcerative colitis occur *most* frequently?
   A. 15–25 year old females
   B. 18–40 year old males and females
   C. 30–50 year old males
   D. 45–60 year old males and females.

345.

346. Ulcerative colitis is *most* prevalent in persons who are:
   A. prone to dietary indiscretions
   B. emotionally disturbed
   C. prone to indigestion
   D. undernourished.

346.

347. The course of ulcerative colitis is essentially:
  A. insidious onset but short duration
  B. acute onset becoming chronic
  C. chronic with acute relapses
  D. acute onset of short duration.

347.

348. The patient is *most* likely to present with:
  A. loss of weight
  B. anaemia
  C. signs of vitamin deficiencies
  D. all of the above.

348.

The doctor visited Anne and carried out a full examination. He asked for certain observations to be made by the nursing staff and arrangements were made for various investigations.

---

349. Which *one* of the following would be the best situation for Anne's bed?
  Near:
  A. the nurses' station
  B. the bathroom
  C. the toilet
  D. the window.

349.

350. Anne's temperature, pulse and respirations were taken and recorded. Her temperature was *most* likely to be:
  A. sub-normal
  B. normal
  C. mildly pyrexial
  D. hyperpyrexial.

350.

351. The number of bowel movements in 24 hours was observed and recorded. These were *most* likely to be in the range of:
  A. 2–5
  B. 6–9
  C. 10–15
  D. 16–20.

351.

352. Which *one* of the following would be present in Anne's stools?
  A. Pus and blood
  B. Fat
  C. Blood and mucus
  D. Altered blood.

352.

A specimen of faecal matter was obtained and sent to the Bacteriological Department for microscopic examination. A specimen of blood was also taken and sent to the Haematology Department for analysis.

353. Which *one* of the following is most likely to be demonstrated on examination of the faeces? The presence of:
    A. Staphylococcus pyogenes
    B. Streptococcus pyogenes
    C. no pathogenic organisms
    D. pertussis bacilli.

353.

354. The haematology report is *most* likely to indicate that Anne is suffering from:
    A. polycythaemia
    B. pernicious anaemia
    C. iron deficiency anaemia
    D. aplastic anaemia.

354.

355. Further diagnostic investigation was requested. This was *most* likely to be:
    A. proctoscopy
    B. sigmoidoscopy
    C. barium enema
    D. digital examination of the rectum.

355.

356. On examination of the bowel mucosa which *one* of the following states would the doctor expect to find?
    A. Necrosis
    B. Thickening and oedema
    C. Gangrene
    D. Suppuration.

356.

Anne was introduced to the other patients in the ward but she was allowed as much privacy as possible to minimise her anxiety and embarrassment.

Medication was prescribed by the doctor in an effort to bring about a reversal of her symptoms.

357. Which *one* of the following should Anne be told to pay particular attention to when carrying out her regular personal hygiene?
    A. Buttocks
    B. Perineum
    C. Shoulders
    D. Heels.

357.

358. Bed rest is important during the acute period of Anne's illness. It should continue until her:
    A. weight begins to increase
    B. dehydration is corrected
    C. number of bowel movements decrease
    D. emotional state has improved.

358.

359. Anne complained of abdominal colic:
    A. continuously
    B. seldom
    C. after food
    D. before a bowel movement.

359.

360. She was encouraged to eat as nourishing a diet as possible. It was *most* important for her diet to contain plenty of:
    A. carbohydrate
    B. roughage
    C. fat
    D. protein.

360.

361. During the acute stage of ulcerative colitis vitamin replacement therapy is necessary. Which *one* of the following groups of vitamins should be given?
    A. A, C and D
    B. B, D and K
    C. B, C and K
    D. C, D and K.

361.

362. The main aim of nursing care and medical treatment is to:
    A. rest the bowel
    B. prepare the patient for surgery
    C. give the patient psychological support
    D. correct weight loss.

362.

363. Oral iron therapy would be prescribed to:
    A. correct blood loss
    B. increase haemoglobin level
    C. increase appetite
    D. to reduce number of stools.

363.

364. Diazepam 2 mg three times a day would be prescribed to: 364.
    A. relieve psychological tension
    B. relieve abdominal discomfort
    C. reduce bowel activity
    D. soothe the mucosa of the bowel.

365. Sulphasalazine (Salazopyrin) was also prescribed. The effect of this drug on   365.
    the bowel is to:
    A. inhibit peristalsis
    B. increase fluid absorption
    C. reduce colic
    D. reduce inflammation.

Anne was also prescribed prednisolone 100 mg daily to be given in divided doses. This would help to reduce the inflammatory process of the disease. Careful observation is necessary during the administration of this drug.

366. The side effects of prednisolone may include: 366.
    A. glycosuria
    B. striae
    C. acne
    D. all of the above.

Anne remained in hospital for a period of six weeks. During this time her general health showed some improvement and the number of stools she passed in each 24 hours was greatly reduced. It was decided to allow her to go home provided she continued to take the prescribed prednisolone, oral iron and vitamin supplements. She was given an appointment to return three weeks later to the medical out-patients clinic.

On Anne's first visit to the clinic she appeared to have maintained her earlier progress. However she was rather reluctant to return to her studies at the university but eventually she agreed to go back at the start of the new term in five weeks' time.

A further appointment was made for Anne to be seen at the clinic but before she could keep it she was re-admitted to the ward. On admission her condition was poor and her diarrhoea very severe.

A surgeon was asked to visit Anne.

367. Surgery for ulcerative colitis can be reversible or irreversible. The purpose of reversible surgery is to:
    A. reduce anaemia
    B. rest the bowel
    C. improve the appetite
    D. alleviate abdominal pain.

367.

368. The *main* reason for undertaking irreversible surgery is to:
    A. give psychological support
    B. prevent complications
    C. improve the quality of life
    D. prevent further weight loss.

368.

369. Which *one* of the following is the *most* common complication of ulcerative colitis?
    A. Septicaemia
    B. Stricture
    C. Perforation
    D. Carcinoma.

369.

In view of Anne's history and present condition it was evident that surgical intervention was necessary.

The surgeon decided to carry out an operation of abdominal perineal resection of the colon. He spoke to both Anne and her parents and fully and carefully explained to them what the surgery would entail and what benefits to Anne could be achieved.

Initially Anne was rather upset at the thought of what was involved but with the support of her parents, nursing and medical staff she overcame most of her fear.

Anne was transferred the following day to a surgical ward.

---

370. The operation of total colectomy with abdomino-perineal excision of rectum results in a permanent:
    A. colostomy
    B. caecostomy
    C. jejunostomy
    D. ileostomy.

370.

371. Pre-operative care was begun five days prior to surgery. Which *one* of the
following would this include?
A. Rectal lavage
B. Milk diet
C. Low residue diet
D. Chest X-ray

371.

372. A course of intestinal antibiotic therapy was prescribed five days prior to
surgery. The purpose of this was to:
A. reduce bowel activity
B. lower the intestinal bacterial count
C. prevent post-operative wound infection
D. prevent post-operative paralytic ileus.

372.

373. A specimen of intravenous blood was sent to the Haematology Department.
It was examined for:
A. haemoglobin levels
B. grouping
C. cross matching
D. all of the above.

373.

374. 24 hours prior to surgery Anne was restricted to fluids only. The reason for
this was to:
A. prevent venous thrombosis
B. prevent post-operative retention of urine
C. reduce colonic peristalsis
D. decrease intestinal residue.

374.

375. On the morning of surgery a nasogastric tube was passed and gentle,
continuous suction of gastric contents was begun. The aim of this was to:
A. prevent vomiting
B. reduce gastric secretion
C. keep the bowel empty
D. maintain fluid balance.

375.

During her period of pre-operative care Anne was visited by a lady
who had received similar surgery for ulcerative colitis some three
years previously and had adjusted successfully to the situation. She
did a great deal to allay many of Anne's not unnatural fears.

On the day of surgery Anne was given routine, pre-operative care.
Her urine was tested, she was bed bathed and dressed in an
operation gown. Her temperature, pulse and respirations were taken
and recorded and she was given her prescribed pre-medication at
the time ordered.

Anne was now ready for surgery and with correct identification, consent form and appropriate records she was taken to the operating theatre.

376. In theatre Anne was given a general anaesthetic and an indwelling catheter was introduced into her bladder. The reason for catheterisation was to prevent:
    A. damage to the urinary bladder during surgery
    B. post-operative retention of urine
    C. urinary tract infection
    D. urethral stricture.

376.

A total colectomy and perineal excision of rectum was carried out. A spout of ileum about 4 cm long was brought through the skin of the abdominal wall on the right side.

377. The *main* purpose of the ileum projection is to:
    A. allow for greater comfort when wearing an ileostomy bag
    B. help to reduce possible excoriation of skin
    C. allow for easier fit of ileostomy bag
    D. allow for easier cleansing.

377.

Post-operative wound care was undertaken according to instructions.

378. Particular attention was paid to the perineal area in order to detect the following. Which *one* would require the *most* immediate action?
    A. Rupture of the wound
    B. Haemorrhage
    C. Infection
    D. Skin irritation.

378.

379. Intravenous fluids were continued post-operatively for 4 days in order to:
    A. correct fluid lost during surgery
    B. correct diminished fluid absorption
    C. prevent urinary retention
    D. prevent vomiting.

379.

380. Aspiration of gastric content via the indwelling nasogastric tube would continue until:
    A. fluid balance is satisfactory
    B. the patient feels like eating
    C. intravenous therapy is discontinued
    D. peristalsis returns.

380.

381. The complication of paralytic ileus may occur. This would be treated by:
    A. continuous gastric suction
    B. intravenous fluids
    C. drugs and physiotherapy
    D. intravenous fluids with continuous gastric suction.

381.

Anne made an uneventful post-operative recovery but she refused to look at her stoma or to show any interest in it. However once her stitches had been removed and her wounds became more comfortable she was encouraged to assist with the care of her stoma. The necessary skin care and application of her ileostomy bags were explained to her. Gradually, helped by the nurses' gentle and understanding approach, she was encouraged to take over the complete care of her ileostomy in preparation for her discharge home.

382. The discharge from the ileostomy:
    A. flows continuously
    B. flows intermittently
    C. is semi-solid
    D. can be controlled.

382.

383. In the immediate post-operative period, the stoma was allowed to discharge:
    A. on to gamgee pads
    B. into a permanent ileostomy bag
    C. into a vacuumed bottle
    D. into a disposable ileostomy bag.

383.

384. To prevent skin irritation Anne was instructed in the use of:
    A. tincture benzoin compound
    B. karaya gum
    C. karaya powder
    D. all of the above.

384.

Anne was now ready to go home. In preparation for discharge she and her mother had a talk with the sister, the stoma therapist and the medical social worker. They were given advice and instruction on several points regarding Anne's future care and well being.

385. Which of the following ileostomy bags would be suitable for Anne?
    A. Permanent ileostomy bag
    B. Disposable ileostomy bag
    C. Deodorising flatus filter bag
    D. Any of the above.

385.

386. Anne should be advised to change the bag:
    A. first thing in the morning
    B. after a meal
    C. before going to bed
    D. at any time.

386.

387. Which *one* of the following pieces of advice should Anne be given with regard to her diet? She should:
    A. eat what she likes
    B. eat plenty of green vegetables
    C. gradually introduce previously troublesome foods
    D. avoid red meat.

387.

388. Anne should be advised to:
    A. limit her fluid intake
    B. increase her fluid intake
    C. avoid drinking coffee
    D. avoid drinking alcohol.

388.

389. Anne should be advised that in future she:
    A. must avoid strenuous exercise
    B. should avoid swimming
    C. should engage in normal healthy exercise and activity
    D. must not have children.

389.

Anne has now been at home for several weeks. While she is still a little apprehensive about the possibility of offensive odour or her bag showing through her clothing, her attitude to life has greatly improved.

Throughout the country there are many people with ileostomies leading full and useful lives. A great deal of help and understanding is given by the Ileostomist Association, which Anne has now joined. She receives their journal regularly and finds it full of helpful advice. Because she is now sharing her experience the magnitude of her problem has been lessened.

Ulcerative colitis answers and explanations

345. **B** While ulcerative colitis can occur at any age the disease is more common in young adults and the early middle aged. It occurs with equal frequency in both men and women.

346. **B** Persons suffering from ulcerative colitis frequently show signs and symptoms of being emotionally disturbed and are often highly-strung and over-protected individuals. The unpleasant nature of the disease may in part be responsible for their emotional disturbance and any stressful situation, for example forthcoming examinations, may result in an acute attack. Dietary indiscretion (A) may cause attacks of diarrhoea but not ulcerative colitis. Undernutrition (D) and indigestion (C) are symptoms of ulcerative colitis not predisposing factors.

347. **C** Ulcerative colitis is insidious in onset and the changes in the bowel mucosa are not apparent in the early stages. Acute relapses occur and eventually the disease becomes chronic.

348. **D** Loss of weight (A) may be due to the patient being afraid to eat in case an acute attack of the disease occurs. Anaemia (B) is due to loss of blood in the stools. Vitamin deficiency (C) occurs because the inflammation of the intestinal mucosa interferes with absorption.

349. **C** Because of the nature of the disease a bed close to the toilet is essential. Many patients find it difficult to use a bed pan and embarrassing to keep asking for a commode.

350. **C** The temperature during an acute attack is usually mildly pyrexial – 37.2°C to 38.3°C. Only rarely would it reach above this level.

351. **C** During an acute attack the number of stools passed in 24 hours is usually in the range of 10–15 although sometimes it may be more.

352. **C** The stools passed are watery containing blood and mucus. The presence of pus in the stool (A) would indicate infection of the colon. Altered blood – melaena (D) – would indicate bleeding from the upper intestinal tract. Fat in the stools (B) is more common in disorders of the biliary tract.

353. **C** Bacteriological examination of a specimen of stool reveals no pathogenic organisms. Staphylococci pyogenes (A) are pus-producing organisms giving rise to such conditions as boils, impetigo and otitis media. Streptococci pyogenes (B) also produce pus and give rise to such conditions as cellulitis and acute tonsillitis. The pertussis bacillus (D) is the infecting organism in whooping cough.

354. **C** The continuous loss of blood in the stools gives rise to iron deficiency anaemia. Polycythaemia (A) is an excessive increase in the number of red blood cells. Pernicious anaemia (B) is due to lack of vitamin B_{12}. Aplastic anaemia (D) is failure of the marrow to produce red blood cells.

355. **B** Diagnostic investigation is by sigmoidoscopy. A sigmoidoscope is a metal tube with a light attached which when passed via the rectum allows visual examination of the lower colon. Proctoscopy (A) and digital examination (D) are too limited. A barium enema (C) is to be avoided because of the risk of causing further inflammation and irritation to the already diseased colon.

356. **B** Examination of the bowel by sigmoidoscopy shows the mucosa to be inflamed with thickening and oedema of the tissue. Gangrene (C) and necrosis (A) would be due to the blood supply to the part being obstructed. Suppuration (D) is the presence of pus.

357. **B** Good general hygiene is essential and while all areas need care the perineum and anal region are at special risk of excoriation due to the frequency of the loose watery stools. Anne should be capable of attending to her own personal hygiene but must be told to report any irritation or soreness. The nurse should however make regular inspections of the perineal and anal areas.

358. **C** Bed rest is essential until the number of bowel movements in 24 hours is reduced. Weight (A) will increase once a suitable diet is introduced. Dehydration (B) can be overcome by fluid replacement. The emotional state (D) can be helped by reassurance and if necessary sedation or tranquillisers.

359. **D** Abdominal colic is present due to bowel activity before a stool is passed.

360. **D** The diet must be high in protein to assist in the repair of body tissue. To reduce the irritation of the mucosa low residue food is given such as eggs, steamed fish and tender meat, e.g. chicken. Greasy foods, raw vegetables and fruit should be avoided. Powdered protein foods such as Casilan can be given with advantage.

361. **C** The vitamins most likely to be deficient are vitamins B, C and K as these are absorbed by the colon. Due to the ulcerative and inflammatory changes in the lining of the colon as well as the excessive diarrhoea the absorption of these vitamins will be greatly reduced.

362. **A** The main aim of treatment is to rest the diseased colon. This is achieved by appropriate medication, diet and bed rest when necessary. In this way the number of daily bowel movements is reduced and the inflammatory state of the colon is reversed.

363. **B** Oral iron therapy is given to restore the low haemoglopy level to normal. Insidious and continuous blood loss from any source results in low haemoglobin levels.

364. **A** Because of the nervous tension that these patients invariably experience, a tranquilliser is often prescribed. The drug in common use is diazepam (Valium) which helps to allay their fear and anxiety.

365. **D** Sulphasalazine is a combination of a sulphonamide with salicylates it is available in 0.5 G tablets and has an anti-inflammatory action. During the acute stage of the illness it is given in doses of 1–2 G four times a day for a period of three weeks.

366. **D** Prednisolone is a steroid and many side effects can occur. The urine should be tested daily for sugar (A). Striae or stretch marks (B) may occur on the abdomen and upper thigh due to fluid retention. Skin eruptions such as acne (C) can also occur.

367. **B** Reversible surgery is carried out in order to put the inflamed colon at complete rest. This is usually done by creating a temporary ileostomy. If the decision is made to perform this type of surgery the period of colonic rest allowed will be from three to six months. After this period it will be possible to assess whether healing of the bowel has taken place and whether normal bowel function can be restored. Surgery is not carried out to reduce anaemia (A) but following surgery the haemoglobin level should be improved. Hopefully at the same time the appetite (C) will increase. Abdominal pain will also be alleviated (D) but this is not the purpose of the operation.

368. **B** Irreversible surgery is mainly carried out to prevent complications. Many patients become less emotional (A) because of the relief of symptoms following surgery and this usually leads to an improved quality of life (C). The appetite will eventually increase and the patient should stop losing weight (D) but these are not the main reasons for surgery.

369. **B** Stricture of the colon (B) is the most common complication. It occurs as a result of the formation of scar tissue and may lead to obstruction. Polypoid changes in the bowel mucosa commonly occur and these may later become malignant (D). Perforation of the colon (C) and septicaemia (A) are possible complications but they are less common.

370. **D** The operation of total colectomy with abdomino-perineal excision of
rectum leaves the patient with a permanent ileostomy. The terminal
portion of the ileum is completely divided and the proximal end is
brought through the skin of the abdominal wall to form an artificial anus
(see Figures).
A, B, C and D are all artificial openings through the abdominal wall to the
skin surface. A colostomy (A) may be a temporary or a permanent
surgical measure with the artificial anus on the proximal side of the
damaged or diseased colon. A caecostomy (B) is an opening into the
caecum, usually performed as a temporary measure in, for example,
acute large bowel obstruction. A jejunostomy (C) is an opening into the
jejunum. It may be performed when there is injury or obstruction of the
small bowel.

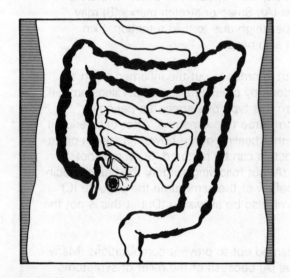

Total colectomy

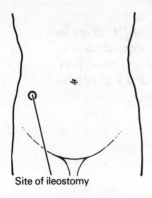

Site of ileostomy

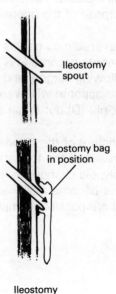

Ileostomy
spout

Ileostomy bag
in position

Ileostomy

371. **C** A low residue diet is given to reduce the content of the bowel and so lessen the risk of faecal spill into the peritoneal cavity during surgery. Rectal lavage (A) is not as a rule prescribed as it may cause further irritation of an already inflamed bowel. A milk diet (B) is not necessary for this patient. A chest X-ray (D) is not routinely required unless there is reason to think it necessary prior to anaesthesia.

372. **B** It is necessary to prepare the intestinal canal by giving a course of an intestinal antibiotic prior to surgery. Lowering the intestinal bacterial count reduces the risk of infection.

373. **D** Because of the severe nature of the surgery to be carried out it is necessary to group and cross match Anne's blood and to estimate her haemoglobin level (A), (B), (C). Haemorrhage is a complication which may occur therefore blood of the correct group and type must be ready should a blood transfusion be required.

374. **D** A 'fluid only' regime given 24 hours prior to surgery further reduces intestinal residue. Venous thrombosis (A) may occur as a complication of lengthy surgery or prolonged post-operative bed rest but a fluid only regime will not prevent this. While a fluid regime of this nature may reduce peristalsis (C) it will have no effect on post-operative retention of urine (B).

375. **C** Nasogastric suction is given prior to surgery to keep the bowel empty. Patients may still vomit (A) even when a nasogastric tube is *in situ*. Gastric secretions (B) are still produced. Fluid balance (D) is maintained by controlled fluid intake during surgery.

376. **A** During lower abdominal surgery the bladder may become damaged as it fills up with urine. If a catheter is passed and left in position on continuous drainage the risk of bladder damage is reduced. Urethral stricture (D) is not a complication of this type of surgery. There is always a risk of urinary tract infection (C) when catheterisation is carried out. Post-operative retention of urine (B) is not always a complication.

377. **B** A 4 cm spout of ileum is brought through the skin to help reduce the possible risk of excoriation of the surrounding skin. The faecal discharge from the ileostomy is rich in enzymes. These have active digestive properties and can attack the skin causing serious skin irritation. The spout will also give a better fit for the ileostomy bag (C), greater comfort (A) and make it easier to clean (D) but the prevention of excoriation is *most* important.

378. **B** Because of the extent of this type of surgery, there is a great risk of post-operative haemorrhage. It is important that such bleeding, should it occur, is detected as soon as possible so that appropriate measures can be taken.
Skin irritation (D) may lead to infection (C) and subsequent breakdown of the wound (A) but with strict asepsis infection should be avoided.

379. **B** The main function of the colon is to absorb water. Because it is now totally removed absorption of water is greatly diminished. Intravenous infusion continues for a minimum of four days to maintain fluid balance and until an adequate oral fluid intake is established.
Intravenous therapy *during* surgery prevents fluid loss (A).

380. **D** Aspiration of gastric content via a nasogastric tube continues until peristalsis returns.

381. **D** Should the complication of paralytic ileus occur it is treated with both intravenous therapy and continuous gastric suction.

382. **A** The discharge from an ileostomy is normally semi-fluid and flows continuously. It is difficult to control but the consistency can be altered by choice of diet and by taking hydrophilic colloids.

383. **D** An adhesive disposable ileostomy bag is used to collect the discharge from the ileostomy spout. If gamgee pads (A) are used the digestive enzymes in the discharge attack the skin. This creates difficulties in achieving a successful seal with either a permanent (B) or a temporary bag. A vacuumed bottle (C) is not used for this type of discharge.

384. **D** Instruction in various methods of keeping the skin surrounding the stoma intact is necessary. Tincture of benzoin compound (A) is painted onto clean dry skin and allowed to dry. This provides a protective surface to which an adhesive ileostomy bag may be attached.
Karaya gum seal (B) forms a close fit round the stoma.
Karaya powder (C) combined with water forms a protective paste. If applied to injured skin it combines with serum exuding from the irritated area to form a dry protective layer.

385. **D** Any of the bags may be used with equally good results. Many types of bag are now produced and a number should be tried out before selecting the one most suitable and convenient for the individual.

386. **A** Although the discharge from the ileostomy cannot be controlled most people find the stoma to be less active first thing in the morning before taking food. Changing the bag at any time (D) is less effective in developing a good routine.

387. **C** It is best to introduce gradually into the diet foods which have been troublesome in the past. In this way problem foods can be eliminated or reduced. Cabbage and other green vegetables (B) may create excessive flatus and more frequent flow from the stoma. It is important that nourishing food, rich in protein and vitamins is eaten. By trial and error Anne should soon establish a well-balanced, nourishing, tasty and varied diet which her ileostomy can cope with.

388. **B** Because of the fluid nature of the stomal discharge an increase in the fluid intake is necessary. While there is no restriction on the type of fluid that can be taken, care should be taken with beverages of an aerated nature such as lemonade or beer which can cause excessive flatus. Alcohol in excess may lead to other problems not associated with her ileostomy but there is no reason why she should avoid alcohol altogether.

389. **C** There is no reason why Anne should curtail her activities because of the ileostomy. Sports and hobbies can be enjoyed to the full. Many women with ileostomies have successful pregnancies therefore there is no reason why Anne should be denied marriage, sex and children.

Nephrotic syndrome

Fiona is six years old. She has a history of repeated urinary tract infections with episodes of enuresis. Recently her mother noticed that Fiona's eyelids were puffy on waking but this puffiness cleared during the day. However, as the day progressed she developed swelling of her legs from the thighs to the ankles. While at school she complained of dizziness. The family doctor was consulted and he arranged Fiona's admission to hospital.

Examination on admission revealed the following: pallor with facial oedema (her eyes were almost closed) and extensive oedema of the abdomen and legs. Her temperature was normal, pulse rate 110 beats per minute, respiration rate 20 per minute and her blood pressure was 110/70 mm Hg.

The following questions (390–438) are all of the multiple choice type. Read the questions and from the possible answers select the ONE which you think is correct. The answers to these questions may be found on pages 97 and 103.

390. Which *one* of the following describes enuresis?
    A. Retention of urine
    B. Suppression of urine
    C. Urinary incontinence in all ages
    D. Urinary incontinence after the age of 3 years.

390.

391. Which *one* of the following could be considered a cause of 'enuresis'?
    A. Delayed neuromuscular maturity
    B. Infection
    C. Emotional disturbance
    D. All of the above.

391.

392. Which *one* of the following best defines oedema?
    A. An increase in body weight
    B. An increase in total body water
    C. Swelling of the tissues
    D. Excess fluid in the interstitial spaces.

392.

393. Which *one* of the following is diagnostic of oedema?
    A. Pitting of the skin
    B. Stretched skin
    C. Dullness of the skin
    D. Loss of elasticity.

393.

394. The average blood pressure in a six-year-old girl is:
    A. 120/75 mm Hg
    B. 112/70 mm Hg
    C. 90/60 mm Hg
    D. 100/65 mm Hg.

394.

Fiona was admitted to the ward where she was allocated a bed in a single cubicle. She was told that for the time being she must stay in bed. Before she got into bed she was weighed. The nurse was told to start recording her fluid intake and output and to take care of her pressure areas.

---

395. Which *one* of the following most accurately describes the reason for isolating Fiona?
    A. She required quietness
    B. To protect other children
    C. To protect Fiona from cross-infection
    D. To provide her with a darkened room.

395.

396. Which *one* of the following most accurately describes the reason for weighing Fiona?
    A. To provide a baseline to determine that she is growing normally
    B. To provide a baseline to determine the results of treatment
    C. To determine the amount of fluid present
    D. To estimate the fluid intake.

396.

397. Fiona was anorexic and her urinary output was low. Which *one* of the following regimes was most likely to be prescribed initially?
    A. Light diet with restricted fluids
    B. Restricted fluids only
    C. Full diet with unlimited fluids
    D. Unlimited fluids only.

397.

398. Which of the following observations and measurements would you consider of primary importance in Fiona's case?
    A. 4-hourly measurement of temperature, pulse and respiration (TPR) and daily measurement of blood pressure
    B. Hourly measurement of blood pressure and 4-hourly TPR
    C. 4-hourly measurement of blood pressure and daily TPR
    D. 4-hourly measurement of blood pressure and TPR.

398.

399. Which *one* of the following most accurately describes the reason for maintaining an accurate fluid chart for Fiona?
   A. To estimate fluid intake and output as an indication of kidney function
   B. To estimate fluid intake only
   C. To ensure that the child drinks regularly
   D. To provide evidence of the frequency of micturition.

399.

400. Which one of the following measures would be taken to prevent formation of pressure and friction sores?
   A. Massage skin
   B. Allow the child to sit out of bed
   C. Change the child's position frequently
   D. Keep the skin clean and dry.

400.

In order to confirm the provisional diagnosis of nephrotic syndrome, investigations of renal function were necessary. These would also provide an assessment of the prognosis. The investigations included urine testing, testing the kidney's ability to concentrate and dilute urine and examination for anatomical abnormalities. A specimen of urine was also taken for biochemical and bacteriological investigations.

---

401. Which *one* of the following methods would be used to obtain a specimen of Fiona's urine for bacteriological examination?
   A. Catheterisation
   B. Normal micturition
   C. 24-hour specimen
   D. Midstream technique.

401.

402. Which *one* of the following abnormal constituents is likely to be present in the urine of a child suffering from nephrotic syndrome?
   A. Sugar
   B. Acetone
   C. Protein
   D. Bile.

402.

403. In Fiona's case which *one* of the following tests is of most significance?
   A. Rothera's test
   B. Clinitest
   C. Esbach's test
   D. Acetest.

403.

The doctor decided to carry out a renal biopsy on Fiona. This examination of renal tissue revealed the type of damage and helped with the assessment of her prognosis. From the results the doctor was able to decide on the best treatment for Fiona. She was prepared for theatre but a general anaesthetic was not required.

404. Which *one* of the following abnormalities would the nurse expect to occur following renal biopsy?
  A. Haematuria
  B. Pyuria
  C. Pain on micturition
  D. Inability to pass urine.

404.

405. After her biopsy Fiona was again confined to bed to prevent complications. Which of the following periods of time would you consider necessary?
  A. Twenty-four hours after return from theatre
  B. Four hours after return from theatre
  C. Until all vital functions are within normal limits and there is no frank haematuria
  D. Two hours after return from theatre.

405.

Fiona was diagnosed as suffering from nephrotic syndrome. She was very oedematous and her urinary output was very low. The doctor prescribed drugs to increase her urinary output.

406. What is the average daily urinary output in a child of six years?
  A. 2000 ml
  B. 1500 ml
  C. 1000 ml
  D. 500 ml.

406.

407. Which of the following drugs would be given to increase Fiona's urinary output?
  A. Spironolactone
  B. Thiazides
  C. Steroids
  D. Mannitol.

407.

408. Which *one* of the following best describes the action of steroids?
  A. They help to maintain water excretion
  B. They interfere with water excretion
  C. They interfere with sodium excretion
  D. They encourage water retention.

408.

409. Which *one* of the following steroids is the drug of choice in the treatment of nephrotic syndrome?
A. Prednisolone
B. Prednisone
C. Dexamethazone
D. Hydrocortisone.

409.

410. Which of the following undesirable effects are associated with steroid treatment?
A. Loss of weight and anorexia
B. Loss of hair and emotional disturbances
C. Redistribution of fat and depletion of body protein
D. Decrease in blood sugar.

410.

411. Children who are not responding to steroids are given cytotoxic drugs. Which one of the following is most usually given?
A. Chlorambucil
B. Daunorubicin
C. Cyclophosphamide
D. Vincristine.

411.

412. Which *one* of the following statements best describes the action of a cytotoxic drug?
A. It destroys all cells
B. It inhibits growth of cells
C. It destroys only abnormal cells
D. It interferes with normal division and development of cells.

412.

413. Diuresis can lead to electrolyte imbalance. Which *one* of the following electrolytes is most likely to be involved?
A. Sodium
B. Potassium
C. Iodine
D. Calcium.

413.

414. Which of the following drugs would be given to prevent electrolyte imbalance?
A. Potassium chloride
B. Slow K
C. Frusemide
D. Sodium chloride.

414.

415. Which *one* of the following diets will be given to Fiona once diuresis has been achieved?
A. Low protein and low salt diet
B. Low protein and normal salt intake
C. High protein and low salt diet
D. High protein and normal salt intake.

415.

The renal biopsy indicated a sclerosing lesion and Fiona's response to treatment was poor. She had frequent relapses and started to show signs of renal failure. It was decided that she could be nursed at home initially. Her parents were given guidance with regard to observations. They were told to contact their family doctor if they were worried.

416. Which of the following signs are indicative of renal failure?   416.
    A. Increased fatigue and lassitude
    B. Increased blood pressure
    C. Decreased urinary output
    D. All of the above.

417. Which of the following should the parents be told to look for?   417.
    A. Appearance of blood in the urine
    B. Increase in oedema with decrease in urinary output
    C. Complaints of headaches
    D. All of the above.

418. When Fiona got home nutrition proved to be a problem. Her appetite was   418.
poor. What diet would you have recommended?
    A. Fluids only
    B. A normal diet for her age
    C. A high carbohydrate diet
    D. A low protein diet.

Fiona's condition deteriorated at home and six weeks after leaving hospital she had to be readmitted for further assessment. It was found that her kidneys were unable to remove toxic material from the blood and it therefore became necessary to find an alternative means of elimination.

419. Which *one* of the following methods would be used to remove toxic   419.
substances from the blood?
    A. Exchange transfusion
    B. Intravenous infusion
    C. Peritoneal dialysis
    D. Diuresis.

420. Which *one* of the following statements best describes a semi-permeable membrane?
    A. A membrane permitting passage of all substances
    B. A membrane permitting passage of water only
    C. A membrane preventing passage of all substances
    D. A membrane permitting passage of certain molecules and preventing that of others.

420.

Fiona was prepared for peritoneal dialysis. This involves passing a catheter through the lower abdominal wall into the peritoneal cavity. Two litres of dialysing fluid are then introduced and are left in the cavity for up to one hour. The fluid is allowed to drain out. This process is repeated and continued until the blood urea levels are near normal. The amount of fluid exchanged in 24 hours varies with the age and condition of the child. It can range from 1 to 10 litres.

421. Which *one* of the following points should the nurse check immediately prior to dialysis?
    A. She has been bathed
    B. She is sedated
    C. Her bladder is empty
    D. She has been weighed.

421.

422. Which of the following solutions would normally be used for peritoneal dialysis?
    A. A hypotonic solution of dextrose
    B. A hypertonic solution of dextrose
    C. A solution of similar electrolyte concentration to extracellular fluid
    D. A solution of similar electrolyte concentration to extracellular fluid but containing no potassium or urea.

422.

423. The solution for dialysis should be at a temperature of:
    A. 31°C
    B. 34°C
    C. 37°C
    D. 40°C

423.

424. Which *one* of the following drugs is added to the dialysing fluid?
    A. Heparin
    B. Antibiotics
    C. Potassium chloride
    D. Steroids.

424.

425. Which of the following observations should the nurse make regularly while dialysis is in progress?
    A. Difficulty in breathing
    B. Evidence of abdominal discomfort
    C. Flow of fluid
    D. All of the above.

425.

426. It is essential to recognise any complications during the dialysis. Which of the following must be monitored?
    A. Temperature, pulse and respirations
    B. Blood sugar level
    C. Plasma protein level
    D. All of the above.

426.

427. What type of diet should Fiona have while on dialysis?
    A. Fluids only
    B. Normal
    C. High protein
    D. Low protein.

427.

Many children are able to undergo peritoneal dialysis while at home. This causes least disturbance to their lives and enables them to continue with school and other normal activities. It is essential that the parents and older children are competent in performing the dialysis. Close liaison between home and hospital is vital. This is achieved through the services of a qualified Sick Children's Nurse who has experience in peritoneal dialysis.

428. Which *one* of the following guidelines should the parents receive regarding home dialysis?
    A. One room in the house should be reconstructed
    B. No special room is required
    C. A separate unit such as a Portacabin should be used
    D. Some minor modification may be required to one room.

428.

429. For which *one* of the following procedures will the parents *not* need to be given special instructions?
    A. Cleaning the room
    B. Handling of sterile equipment
    C. Storage of sterile equipment
    D. Disposal of used fluid.

429.

430. Which of the following events occurring during dialysis would indicate   430.
complications?
A. Cloudiness of returned fluid
B. Inadequate amount of returned fluid
C. The child complains of dizziness
D. All of the above.

431. Which of the following specimens should the home nurse obtain at regular   431.
intervals?
A. Returned fluid for pathology
B. Returned fluid for bacteriology and biochemistry
C. Swab from catheter for bacteriology and returned fluid for pathology
D. Swab from catheter for bacteriology and returned fluid for bacteriology
and biochemistry.

Fiona continued to attend school. The teachers had to be informed
of her treatment and what symptoms she was likely to complain of.
They also had to be told what action they should take if the child
felt unwell.

432. In which of the following school activities could Fiona participate?   432.
A. Physical education
B. Classroom activities only
C. Classroom and limited playground activities
D. Unlimited activities.

433. Which of the following symptoms is Fiona likely to complain of?   433.
A. Listlessness
B. Dizziness
C. Headaches
D. All of the above.

Fiona's condition was frequently assessed and the clinical features
and biochemical tests indicated that peritoneal dialysis had failed to
remove excess urea from the blood. The doctor decided to use the
more effective treatment – haemodialysis. This involves the insertion of one end of a loop of tubing into an artery and the other into a
vein, usually in the patient's arm. When dialysis is not being carried
out blood flows uninterrupted between the artery and the vein. To
carry out haemodialysis the tube is clamped and taken apart in the
middle. The arterial end is connected to the arterial tube on a kidney

machine and the machine then takes on the functions of a normal kidney. The blood passes through the machine and flows out through the venous tube of the machine which is attached to the venous end of the shunt (see Figure).

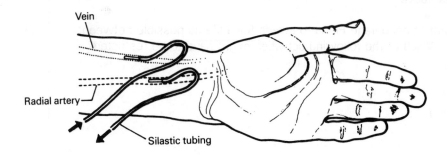

434. Which *one* of the following best describes the advantage of haemodialysis?
    A. It is only carried out twice weekly
    B. There is no danger of peritonitis
    C. Biochemical correction can be achieved in a shorter time than with peritoneal dialysis
    D. It causes least disturbance to the child.

434.

435. Which *one* of the following diets would Fiona be given during haemodialysis?
    A. Normal
    B. Normal without added salt or extra fluid
    C. High protein
    D. High protein, low salt.

435.

436. Which *one* of the following methods would you use to ensure that the child can feed herself during haemodialysis?
    A. Loosen the restraint on the cannulated arm
    B. Give her minced food and a spoon
    C. Cut up her food and provide her with suitable cutlery
    D. Give her the food and encourage her to cut it up herself.

436.

Fiona adapted fairly easily to the frequent sessions of haemodialysis. However chronic illness has disturbing effects on the family and this is often reflected by the child's attitude and behaviour.

437. Which of the following people could play an important part in helping Fiona and her family?
    A. Psychiatrist
    B. Clinical psychologist
    C. Medical social worker
    D. All of the above.

437.

438. It is important to encourage Fiona to live as full a life as possible between treatments. Which of the following activities might have to be restricted?
    A. Running
    B. Cycling
    C. Skipping
    D. Swimming.

438.

Nephrotic syndrome answers and explanations

390. **D** Enuresis or bedwetting is normal during the first two or three years of life. However, by the time the child is 2½–3 years old he should have achieved urethral sphincter control. Failure to achieve that control leads to enuresis.

391. **D** All of the options could be considered a cause of 'enuresis'. In Fiona's case it is likely that infection of the renal tract was the cause.

392. **D** Tissue fluid balance is maintained by the counteraction of two pressures: blood pressure and the osmotic pressure of plasma protein. This is achieved by the following processes:
1. At the arterial end of the capillaries the blood pressure is greater than the osmotic pressure. As a result fluid is forced through the capillary walls into the tissue spaces.
2. At the venous end the osmotic pressure is greater than the blood pressure and fluid is therefore drawn into the capillary.
Normally these two opposing factors keep a steady balance of fluid in the tissues. Any factor which disturbs this equilibrium may lead to oedema. Oedema is said to be present when there is excess fluid in the interstitial spaces. For example, sodium and water retention leads to increased blood pressure and loss of protein in the urine (proteinuria). This leads to a decrease in plasma protein (hypoproteinaemia) and therefore decreases osmotic pressure. Fluid then collects and stagnates in the interstitial spaces. See Figure.

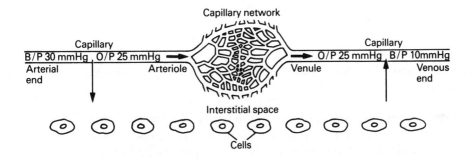

393. **A** To identify the presence of oedema, digital pressure is applied to the swollen area. Removal of digital pressure leaves a characteristic indentation or pitting of the tissues.

394. **C**

395. **C** Prevention of cross-infection is important for all patients, but infection in children suffering from nephrotic syndrome can lead to circulatory disturbance and shock. This is believed to be due to a reduction in the volume of the circulating blood (hypovolaemia) resulting from loss of protein in the urine and fluid loss from the blood into the tissues. As a result of the protein loss there may also be a decreased ability to manufacture and retain antibodies. It is therefore desirable to provide some isolation initially to prevent cross-infection, though many units do not advocate such measures except where the child is on immunosuppressive drug therapy.

396. **B** Fiona must be weighed on admission to provide a baseline to help determine the results of her treatment. Subsequently daily weighing is usually required to determine increase or decrease in weight as a result of either retention of fluid or successful diuresis.

397. **B** Since Fiona is anorexic it is probably better to give her fluids only initially. As she has oedema it is probable that there is damage to her kidneys. Until this is investigated her fluid intake should be restricted to about one litre in 24 hours. This can be given as 500 ml of milk and 500 ml of fruit juice.

398. **A** Temperature, pulse and respiration are measured and recorded 4-hourly. A rise in temperature, pulse and respiration rates might indicate an underlying infection. The breathing rate, rhythm and depth should be observed to identify the accumulation of fluid in the pleural cavity (pleural effusion). The blood pressure is usually measured once a day since it is generally normal. However, transient hypertension may be present, particularly where there are definite lesions of the renal glomeruli.

399. **A** It is essential to maintain an accurate fluid intake and output chart. This is to ensure an adequate intake of fluid, to help calculate fluid requirements and to provide a visual means of determining the degree of diuresis.

400. **C** In order to prevent the formation of pressure sores it is important that the child's position is changed frequently. Since Fiona is on bed rest this is the responsibility of the nurse. Restriction of activity will be based on the amount of oedema present. If the oedema is mild, the child may be allowed out of bed for short periods (B), but this will be at the discretion of the doctor. Even in excessive oedema it is often more comfortable to sit out of bed for a little while. It is always important to keep the skin clean and dry (D).

401. **D** A specimen of urine sent for bacteriological examination should be uncontaminated. It is however more usual to obtain a midstream specimen of urine than to catheterise, since catheterisation is not without danger. In Fiona's case the bacteriological examination is necessary because of her history of urinary tract infection.

402. **C** Proteinuria is definitive of nephrosis. Qualitative tests for protein may show a +++ or ++++ reaction and this could be equated quantitatively as being equivalent to 300–1000 mg/100 ml. (A test for the presence of a substance is termed 'qualitative'. A test for the amount of a substance is termed 'quantitative'.)

403. **C** An Esbach quantitative protein test is performed to determine the amount of protein present in the urine. Acidified urine is put into an Esbach's albuminometer and mixed with Esbach's reagent. It is allowed to stand for 24 hours and the protein will precipitate. The level of the precipitate is read on the tube's scale and is recorded as grammes per litre (g/l). Rothera's and Acetest (A and D) are tests for ketones. Clinitest (B) is a test for sugar.

404. **A** Haematuria tends to be transient following renal biopsy. Perirenal bleeding may occur in a few cases. It is therefore essential that the child is carefully observed during the 24 hours following renal biopsy.

405. **C** The child is usually kept on bedrest for 24 hours following renal biopsy but the most important deciding factors are the return of vital functions to normal limits and the absence of frank haematuria.

406. **C** Urinary output in a six-year-old child is within the range of 900 ml to 1300 ml in 24 hours.

407. **C** Corticosteroids induce remissions in patients with minimal lesions of the kidney glomerulus. Diuresis generally occurs one to two weeks after therapy starts. This is followed by a reduction in the oedema.

408. **A** Corticosteroids permit many biochemical reactions to proceed at optimal rates. They help to maintain the capacity of the nephrons to excrete water.

409. **B** Prednisone is the drug of choice. It has the best anti-inflammatory action and sodium and water retention is less than with other steroids.

410. **C** Corticosteroids influence the release of liver glycogen and can cause hyperglycaemia. High doses result in redistribution of fat with increased deposition in the face and abdominal regions. They also affect protein metabolism and can cause severe muscle wasting and osteoporosis.

411. **C** Cyclophosphamide is usually used. Oedema and proteinuria take longer to clear than with other drugs but relapses are fewer.

412. **D** Cytotoxic substances are efficient in killing tumour cells. However, since they interfere with DNA synthesis they may also kill healthy cells.

413. **B** Hypokalaemia (low potassium level in the blood) is the most common
and   side-effect of diuretics. If untreated this may lead to metabolic alkalosis.
414. **B** For this reason a supplement of potassium is prescribed when treatment with diuretics is required. To prevent sudden overload the potassium is given in a slow releasing form (Slow K).

415. **C** Since protein is continually being lost it is important to replace it as far as possible by giving a high protein diet. At first this should be salt-free but once diuresis is achieved some salt can be given in the diet without producing oedema.

416. **D** Lack of energy with increased fatigue on exertion are the usual observable signs. Initially they are slight and any gradual change in behaviour is hard to detect. The lassitude is often associated with anaemia. The blood pressure is often elevated and may be associated with uraemia. In some cases the rise in blood pressure is due to the action of renin, which is secreted by the ischaemic kidney in response to decreases in blood pressure.

417. **D** Blood will appear in the urine (A) when the glomeruli are affected and this is an indication of deterioration. Severe headaches (C) are symptomatic of raised blood pressure. An increase in oedema (B) indicates increased protein loss. As more nephrons are affected less urine will be produced (B).

418. **B** In the early stages of renal failure no special diet is necessary. The aim of dietary intake is to provide adequate amounts of protein and calories to meet growth and activity needs. With further deterioration of renal function, dietary adjustments are made to limit the amount of solutes passing to the kidneys. A protein intake of 2 to 3 g per kilogram of body weight is desirable to make good the protein loss, provided the blood urea levels remain normal. If they become elevated it may be necessary to restrict protein intake (D).

419. **C** In peritoneal dialysis the patient's peritoneum provides a semi-permeable
and   membrane. A dialysing fluid is run into the peritoneal cavity which serves
420. **D** as the dialysis bath. When the peritoneal cavity is filled with the dialysing fluid an exchange of solutes takes place across the peritoneal membrane between the plasma and the fluid in the peritoneal cavity. Since the membrane is semi-permeable it will permit the passage of certain molecules only.

421. **C** The most important point for the nurse to check immediately prior to dialysis is that the bladder is empty. In the empty state the bladder is a pelvic organ; when full it becomes an abdominal organ. Unless the bladder is empty there is danger of bladder injury during catheter insertion.
Cleanliness of the child (A) is important to minimise infection. Full aseptic technique must be observed during the insertion of the catheter. It is helpful if the child is calm and sedated prior to the insertion of the catheter. If the child is conscious and restless sedation should be given (B). Despite the local anaesthetic this procedure tends to be painful.

422. **D** The standard solution used for dialysis has an electrolyte concentration similar to that of extracellular fluid but contains no potassium or urea. On occasion hypertonic solutions with higher concentrations of glucose (4–7 per cent) are used in an attempt to relieve oedema or circulatory overload. The solution acts as an osmotic force and increases the rate of filtration.

423. **C** The solution should be at body temperature (37°C). This is more comfortable and is also believed to increase the transfer of urea across the peritoneal membrane. Introduction of cold fluid (A and B) would lead to a fall in body temperature.

424. **A** Heparin is added to prevent fibrin formation around the catheter tip. The small amount of heparin is not sufficient to interfere with the systemic blood clotting mechanism. (B) Antibiotics are not given routinely but are reserved for specific peritoneal infection. (C) Potassium chloride may be given to titrate against the potassium loss. (D) Steroids are not added to the dialysing fluid since they are best absorbed by either oral or intravenous routes.

425. **D** It is particularly important to observe the flow of fluid (C) to ensure that most if not all of it is returned. Discomfort or pain (B) may be present due to increasing volume of fluid in the peritoneal cavity. This could press on the diaphragm and cause difficulty in breathing (A).

426. **D** A variety of complications may occur during peritoneal dialysis. These include:
Hyperglycaemia due to diffusion of the infused glucose into the extracellular fluid. This is the reason for observing the blood sugar level (B).
Hyperproteinaemia due to protein loss during repeated dialysis. This is the reason for observing the plasma protein level (C).
There is a risk of peritonitis which can be recognised by tenderness of the abdomen, a rise in body temperature, pulse rate and breathing rate (A).

427. **C** A high protein diet is given to replace the protein lost due to repeated peritoneal dialysis. There is no need to restrict fluid intake.

428. **D** Minimal modification is required but a wash-hand basin should be available and extra cupboard accommodation and shelves may be required.

429. **D** To prevent infection it is essential that the parents should be able to perform the procedure efficiently and under aseptic conditions. They will need to be given special instructions for (A), (B) and (C) but no special instructions are needed for the disposal of the fluid.

430. **D** All three options are signs of possible complications. If the returned fluid is cloudy (A) this indicates infection is present. A feeling of dizziness might be due to a fall in blood pressure (C). It is also important for Fiona's parents to weigh her every morning with the fluid out of the abdomen. This will give an early indication should any fluid retention occur. This would be a serious complication resulting in increased blood pressure, headaches, visual disturbances, vomiting and convulsions.

    Her temperature should also be recorded regularly as an increase would indicate infection and a decrease would indicate shock.

431. **D** The returned fluid should be analysed regularly by the biochemist and tested for micro-organisms by the bacteriologist. Bacteriological examination of wound and catheter must be carried out to identify pathogenic organisms and to test for sensitivity.

432. **C** Classroom and limited playground activities are probably most suitable but the child will know her limitations. Some days she may feel able to take part in the usual playtime activities while on other days she may feel more lethargic.

433. **D**

434. **C** Six hours of haemodialysis achieves essentially the same degree of biochemical correction as twenty-four hours of peritoneal dialysis.

435. **B** Generally there is no need to restrict the diet during dialysis. However sometimes a diet containing no added salt or extra fluid is prescribed.

436. **C** It is important to allow Fiona to be as independent as possible. It is not easy to cut food into small pieces with one hand and so the nurse should do this for her. She should then ensure that the plate and suitable cutlery are placed in such a position that the child can feed herself without difficulty.

437. **D** Generally children adapt readily to haemodialysis but many show signs of emotional disturbance. Tensions in the home are created by the additional strain imposed on all the family and contribute to the child's stress. Parents as well as children have to be helped to face the problems of chronic illness. In any haemodialysis programme it is therefore important to have within the team a psychiatric consultant (A), a clinical psychologist (B) and a medical social worker (C) as well as the home nurse. Each has an important part to play. The medical social worker will help with any social or economic problem; the clinical psychologist will help the child and family to recognise and overcome problems; the psychiatrist will help in treating depression. The home nurse acts as a link between all and gives support during the special procedures to both the child and her parents.

438. **D** There is no need to restrict Fiona's activity between treatments. If she had an external shunt then swimming would not be allowed.

Case history on urinary calculi

James Rushton was a 19-year-old student, living in the university hall of residence. His widowed mother and 12-year-old sister lived in the South of England, and James looked forward to his infrequent visits home. His health had always been excellent, so following two episodes of loin pain and haematuria, he was worried and went to see his general practitioner.

True false questions

The following questions (439–457) consist of a number of statements, some of which are true and some of which are false. Consider each statement and decide whether you think it is true or false. You can indicate your answer by writing T for true or F for false in the right hand margin beside each statement.

The answers to these questions may be found on pages 112 to 115.

On his initial visit to the surgery his doctor was likely to undertake the following investigations:

439. A rectal and abdominal examination. | 439.

440. A detailed medical history. | 440.

441. A general examination and urinalysis. | 441.

442. Collection of blood for biochemical analysis. | 442.

The general practitioner referred James to the out-patient clinic of the local hospital to confirm his urinary calculi. He was given an appointment for the following week.

In out-patients the following tests were likely to be carried out:

443. A mid-stream specimen of urine. | 443.

444. Retrograde pyelography. | 444.

445. Twenty-four hour urine for urea and electrolytes. | 445.

446. Intravenous pyelogram.	446.
447. Blood for serum calcium levels.	447.
448. Twenty-four hour urine collection for calcium excretion.	448.
449. Blood for uric acid level.	449.
450. Blood for urea and electrolytes.	450.
451. Blood for serum acid phosphate.	451.
452. Early morning urine for cystine level.	452.
453. Twenty-four hour urine collection for protein levels.	453.

The following statements (454–457) refer to renal colic.

454. An impacted stone will cause sudden and severe loin pain.	454.
455. Pain radiation *is not* related to the level of the obstruction.	455.
456. Pain caused by a partially obstructing stone may be aggravated by drinking.	456.
457. Pain *is not* associated with nausea and vomiting.	457.

Multiple choice questions

The following questions (458–479) are all of the multiple choice variety. Read the question and from the four possible answers select the ONE which you think is correct.

458. The most common crystalloid which forms renal calculi is:
    A. cystine
    B. calcium
    C. xanthine
    D. uric acid.

    458.

459. The formation of renal calculi may be enhanced by:
    A. antibiotics
    B. cytotoxic drugs
    C. diuretic drugs
    D. corticosteroids.

    459.

460. Calculi may be formed if there is:
    A. prolonged antibiotic therapy
    B. excess fluid intake
    C. immobilisation
    D. over-activity.

    460.

461. A stone which is impacted at the pelvi-ureteric junction gives rise to pain which is felt in the:
    A. abdomen
    B. groin
    C. loin
    D. thigh.

    461.

462. One of the first signs of a sudden impaction of a ureteric calculus is:
    A. infection
    B. hydronephrosis
    C. renal infarction
    D. haematuria.

    462.

Following his visit to the out-patient department James returned to his hall of residence to await the results of the tests. One evening he went to a party given by some student friends. In the early hours of the morning, he complained of severe loin pain and nausea, and started perspiring heavily. As a result his friends called an ambulance and he was admitted to hospital.

463. Following admission, one of the most important procedures that the nurse will undertake is:
    A. the collection of a twenty-four hour urine specimen
    B. to test all urine for specific gravity
    C. to sieve all specimens of urine
    D. to save all urine for inspection.

463.

464. A specimen of urine will be tested daily for:
    A. pH
    B. ketones
    C. blood
    D. glucose.

464.

465. After admitting James, the nursing staff *must* inform:
    A. the university
    B. his mother
    C. neither
    D. both.

465.

466. If his mother wished to visit him, but could not return home, she would be referred to the:
    A. university
    B. medical staff
    C. nursing officer
    D. nearest hotel.

466.

467. Should she be unable to visit, it is preferable that information will be given to her on the telephone by the:
    A. ward clerk
    B. ward sister
    C. nursing officer
    D. consultant-in-charge.

467.

468. James' daily fluid intake should be:
    A. 1–1½ litres
    B. 2–2½ litres
    C. 3–3½ litres
    D. 4–4½ litres.

468.

469. The doctor may order Pro-Banthine to be given to:
    A. increase fluid output
    B. relax smooth muscle
    C. decrease fluid output
    D. relax skeletal muscle.

469.

470. One of the most important adverse reactions to watch for when giving Pro-Banthine is:
    A. bradycardia
    B. urinary retention
    C. diarrhoea
    D. postural hypotension.

470.

471. The doctor prescribed an analgesic to relieve James' pain. Which of the following would be most suitable?
    A. Fortral tablets
    B. Omnopon injection
    C. Distalgesic tablets
    D. Pethidine injection.

471.

472. Samples of blood for urea and electrolyte levels will be collected. The normal range for blood urea is:
    A. 1–2 millimole per litre
    B. 4–5 millimole per litre
    C. 7–8 millimole per litre
    D. 10–11 millimole per litre.

472.

Because James' intravenous pyelogram had demonstrated ureteric calculi, and since his symptoms had not subsided, the consultant decided to proceed with surgery.

473. Ureteric calculi may be removed by:
    A. litholapaxy
    B. pyelolithotomy
    C. partial nephrectomy
    D. uretero lithotomy.

473.

474. On preparing James for operation, it is the *nurse's* responsibility to ensure that:
    A. the operation site is marked
    B. an identiband is in place
    C. a consent form is signed
    D. the blood is grouped and cross-matched.

474.

475. Immediately before going to the operating theatre, James would have:
    A. his urea and electrolytes estimated
    B. a specimen of urine tested
    C. an abdominal X-ray
    D. his blood pressure estimated.

475.

476. On James' return from theatre, the nurse's *primary* concern was to:
    A. check the wound site
    B. record the blood pressure
    C. maintain a clear airway
    D. connect the drainage bag.

476.

477. Observations of blood pressure and pulse were recorded:
    A. whenever necessary
    B. half-hourly
    B. once only
    D. as instructed.

477.

478. Which of the following positions would James be nursed in during the first twenty-four hours?
    A. Recumbent
    B. Lateral
    C. Upright
    D. The most comfortable.

478.

479. Fluids were allowed when:
    A. bowel sounds returned
    B. vomiting ceased
    C. consciousness returned fully
    D. urine was passed.

479.

True false questions

The following questions (480–487) consist of a number of statements, some of which are true and some of which are false. Consider each statement and decide whether you think it is true or false.

480–483. Intravenous fluids may be given post-operatively. The fluid of choice may be:

480. normal saline 0.9%
481. dextrose 0.18%, saline 0.9%
482. Hartmann's solution
483. Ringer's solution.

480.
481.
482.
483.

484–487. The intravenous infusion may be discontinued on the doctor's instructions, when:

484. bowel sounds have returned
485. urine has been passed
486. there is no nausea or vomiting
487. wound drainage is minimal.

484.
485.
486.
487.

The following questions (488–491) are all of the multiple choice type.

488. James was encouraged to get up within:
   A. 1–2 days
   B. 3–4 days
   C. 5–6 days
   D. 7–8 days.

488.

489. His sutures were removed in:
   A. 4–5 days
   B. 7–8 days
   C. 10–11 days
   D. 12–13 days.

489.

After approximately 10 days, James was allowed home. On discharge he was given an out-patient appointment.

490. When he returned to out-patients which one of the following tests was he
most likely to have repeated?
A. Intravenous pyelogram
B. Serum calcium
C. Abdominal X-ray
D. Urea and electrolytes.

490.

491. James was advised to make changes in his diet. They were likely to be in
the form of:
A. increased dairy products and decreased fluid intake
B. increased protein products and increased fluid intake
C. decreased diary produce and increased fluid intake
D. decreased protein products and decreased fluid intake

491.

Urinary calculi answers and explanations

439. **False** An abdominal examination will be relevant. However rectal examination should not be necessary as the haematuria is unlikely to be caused by enlargement of the prostate glad in view of the patient's age.

440. **True** It is important to obtain all relevant facts

441. **True** Urinalysis will detect haematuria (microscopic) and proteinuria, whilst the general examination will indicate the state of health.

442. **False** The general practitioner is unlikely to collect blood for analysis at this stage as no definite diagnosis has yet been made.

443. **True** A mid-stream specimen of urine is usually examined to detect any underlying infection.

444. **False** Retrograde pyelography is not undertaken in the out-patient department as a general anaesthetic is required with cystoscopy and serial X-rays.

445. **False** This is not relevant in this particular disease. It is used in the diagnosis of parenchymal diseases.

446. **True** This examination can be done in the out-patient department. It will demonstrate the presence and function of kidneys and *may* show calculi and filling defects. If calculi are present it will show their position establishing whether they are renal (in the kidney) or ureteric (in the ureters).

447. **True** One sample of each may be taken as a guide to further investigations. Three fasting serial blood samples and three serial urine calcium level estimations are required to detect hyper-parathyroidism.

448. **True** James was given a provisional diagnosis of renal calculi. One of the possible causes is hyperparathyroidism in which condition there is increased excretion of calcium by the kidneys which may lead to development of calculi.

449. **False** This would be more relevant in age groups when gout may be present as a pre-disposing cause in which case the uric acid level would be elevated.

450. **True** This will indicate his present state of renal function.

451. **False** A high serum acid phosphate level is indicative of malignant change, but this is usually associated with prostatic enlargement.

452. **True** Cystine is a metabolic substance which may be precipitated in the urine (cyseinuria). This is a metabolic disorder which is one cause of renal stones. A single test of an early morning urine specimen would demonstrate its presence.

453. **False** This test will only be carried out if renal damage is suspected.

454. **True** Yes it will. An impacted stone will obtruct the ureter and cause waves of peristalsis and severe colicky pain.

455. **False** This pain usually radiates downwards from the loin to the groin but its level may help to determine the site of stone.

456. **True** Renal colic may be aggravated by drinking. This increases the urinary flow, causing movement of the stone, so increasing the risk of impaction.

457. **False** Renal colic is often associated with nausea and vomiting.

458. **B** 90 per cent of all calculi have a calcium base. The remaining 10 per cent may be of either cystine (A) or uric acid (D).

459. **D** Corticosteroids break down the protein matrix of bone, causing calcium to be released into the urine. This leads to a pre-disposition to calculi formation.

460. **C** Immobilisation results in osteoporosis (or thinning of the bone), excess calcium is released into the blood stream and this is excreted by the kidney leading to the formation of renal calculi.

461. **C** A stone which is impacted at the pelvi-ureteric junction gives rise to pain in the loin as this is the point at which the ureter leaves the kidney. If the stone is in the ureter proper, pain may be felt in the iliac fossa, the groin or the external genitalia or the thigh (A), (B), (D).

462. **D** Haematuria (D) presents first. As tissue is damaged infection (A) may superimpose, and hydronephrosis (B) may occur if the obstruction is complete. Infarction (C) is unlikely.

463. **C** This is one procedure the nurse can undertake straight away. She may obtain gravel which the laboratory can then use to identify the crystalloid form; this may help in diagnosing the cause of the calculi.

464. **C** Gravel or an impacted calculus will probably cause either microscopic or macroscopic haematuria. A ward-based urine test is a quick way of detecting this. A follow-up test would be the examination of a mid-stream specimen of urine for red blood cells.

465. **C** James was over the age of consent, and relatives and places of work should only be informed with his agreement.

466. **C** If overnight accommodation was available, the nursing officer would arrange it in conjunction with the ward sister, home wardens or personnel officer. If not, she might refer her to a hotel or to the social worker for advice.

467. **B** Initially the best person to give information to Mrs Rushton and to reassure her was the ward sister. She might also wish to speak to one of the doctors in charge as well as to her son.

468. **C** This is approximately 6 pints of fluid, an amount that most men manage to drink without too much trouble. It dilutes urine, aids diuresis and the passage of gravel.

469. **B** Pro-Banthine is given orally in order to relax the smooth muscle.

470. **B** Pro-Banthine is an atropine-type drug which causes urinary retention but may also cause hypertension, tachycardia and constipation.

471. **D** Pethidine takes effect within 15 minutes, it peaks in 1 hour and is excreted well. It is less toxic than morphine, has anticholinergic effects and therefore relaxes the smooth muscle of the ureter.

472. **B** The normal range for blood urea is 4–5 millimoles per litre.

473. **D** Lithotomy literally means removal of a stone. Uretero lithotomy is the removal of a stone from the ureter (D). Litholapaxy (A) means crushing a stone within the bladder. Pyelolithotomy (B) is the surgical removal of a stone from the renal pelvis. Nephrectomy (C) means the removal of a kidney.

474. **B** The nurse must see that the identiband is in place. The other items listed are the doctor's responsibility, although the nurse may be asked to check them.

475. **C** An abdominal X-ray will indicate the site of the calculus at the time of operating. This will make it easier for the surgeon to choose an accurate point of entry into the ureter. The other tests should have been carried out already.

476. **C** All the points listed are important, but the nurse's primary concern is to keep the airway clear.

477. **D** The frequency of the observations will depend upon the patient's condition, and this should be assessed by the medical staff before he leaves theatre. The doctor should instruct the nursing staff regarding the observations he wishes to be made.

478. **D** Any of the first three positions may be used, but it is more important for the patient to be in a position which is comfortable.

479. **C** Oral fluids will be given when he is fully conscious, and will be increased when bowel sounds return and vomiting ceases.

480. **True** ⎤ If the reason for giving IV fluid post-operatively is to increase the flow of urine through the ureter either normal saline or a dextrose
481. **True** ⎟ and saline solution may be used. These are both physiologically normal solutions.
482. **False** ⎟ Hartmann's and Ringer's solutions both contain added electrolytes and would only be used to correct electrolyte imbalance.
483. **False** ⎦

484. **True** ⎤ The return of bowel sounds and the cessation of nausea and vomiting indicate that the intestinal tract has returned to normal, and
485. **False** ⎟ that intravenous fluids are no longer necessary. Wound drainage will decrease within 3–5 days and urine should be passed normally
486. **True** ⎟ within 24 hours.
487. **False** ⎦

488. **A** It is advisable to start mobilisation as soon as possible in order to minimise post-operative complications.

489. **B** Seven to eight days (B) is the most probable time range. Four to five days (A) would be too soon and ten to fifteen days (C) or twelve to thirteen days (D) would apply only if the patient had poor healing capacity due to age or undernourishment.

490. **A** A repeat intravenous pyelogram may be undertaken to check the state of the urinary tract and excretory function, as well as the presence of any other calculi.

491. **C** An excess of dairy produce which is rich in calcium may increase calcium deposition and a low fluid intake may result in stasis. These are both pre-disposing factors in the formation of calculi.